Principles of Safe Practice in
The Perioperative Environment
CONTENTS

Revised November 1998
Published by National Association of Theatre Nurses
Copyright © 1998 by NATN
ISBN 0 9518380 67

National Association of Theatre Nurses, Daisy Ayris House, 6 Grove Park Court,
Harrogate, HG1 4DP Tel: +44 (0)1423 508079 Fax: +44(0)1423 531613
www.natn.org.uk

Designed and printed by Maxiprint, Clifton Moor, York, England YO30 4XF
www.maxiprint.co.uk

SMC

This document was revised by the
National Association of Theatre Nurses' Education Committee.
The publication was designed, compiled and assembled by the Association's Editorial
Board, members of Council, reviewers and Headquarters staff.

NATN would like to thank and acknowledge the immense effort invested in the
production of the document by everybody who has contributed in any way. We feel it
is a significant advance on the previous editions and hope that it becomes a major
addition to the reference tools of operating departments.

Principles of Safe Practice in The Perioperative Environment

Environment - *Section 1*

Reviewers

Pat Bunch RGN BSc (Hons)
Theatre and Outpatients Services Manager
The Berkshire Independent Hospital

Vi Haddow RGN PGDip
Associate Director Private Healthcare
Lambeth, Southwark and Lewisham Health Authority

Jane Reid RGN DPSN BSc(Hons) PGCEA
Senior Lecturer Critical Care
Institute of Health and Community Studies
Bournemouth University
Bournemouth

Principles of Safe Practice in
The Perioperative Environment

Environment - *Section 1*

FIRE

Introduction

It is essential for all operating theatre departments to demonstrate a commitment to the Health & Safety at Work Act 1974 by having clearly defined up to date policies and procedures relating to fire prevention in order to maintain safety within the department for patients and staff. It is recommended that policies and procedures are considered in conjunction with the NATN Risk Assessment Guide (NATN 1995).

NATN has listed the necessary documentation needed to research and develop local procedures along with the main recommendations that ought to be considered as part of the overall document:

BIBLIOGRAPHY

Strategy

Fire Services Act 1947

Fire Precautions Act 1984

Fire Safety and Safety at Places of Sport Act (amended Fire Precautions Act 1974)

Health and Safety at Work Act 1974

Registered Homes Act 1984

Buildings Act 1984

DOH 1987 Directory of Fire Document. (ISBM 0113211082)

NHS Estates 1991 Health Building Notes 26 Operating Department. London, HMSO

National Policies

Fire Precautions in NHS Premises
Fire Code 1987 HC 8724, November
Fire Precautions (Workplace) Regulations 1977 ISBN 0-11-064738-6

Regulations

Building Regulations 1985
Local Authority Regulations

There should be a departmental policy which incorporates all of the above plus organisational policies drawn up in conjunction with the fire officer and users. This should then be approved by the relevant committee for Health and Safety and ratified by the Executive Board of the hospital or health care organisation.

REFERENCES

HM (86) 17 - Fire Precautions

Health Building Note 2025

HTM - Fire Precautions

HTM 2022 Medical Gases

Alarm and Call systems HTM 2010 DOH HMSO

IEE Wiring and Regulations 16th Ed BS7671 1992 ISBN 0-85296-557-5

Portable Electrical Appliances HSE Guidance PM 32

DOH 1987 Fire Code - Directory of Fire Documents. DOH, ISBN 0113211082, HMSO

NATN 1995 Risk Assessment Guide (RAG). Harrogate

Recommendations for Consideration When Devising a Local Policy

a. As part of planning a new complex or refurbishment of a theatre suite the project team should consult with the specialist personnel.

b. All units must take sensible precautions against fire in consultation with fire safety officer or specialist fire prevention officer.

c. It is essential that there is a nominated fire officer.

d. Advice and assistance of the chief fire officer of the local fire authority should be sought when defining policies and procedures in hospitals and other health premises.

e. Policies should stipulate that all staff attend a fire lecture and practice on **not less** than one occasion per year.

f. There should be a register of attendance, signed by participants.

g. It is essential that there is a well developed procedure for evacuation and this should be part of the induction course for newly appointed staff.

h. Evacuation procedures for patients and staff should be practised on **not less** than one occasion per year.

i. Risk management requires commitment and awareness by all staff, for example the necessity of keeping fire exits clear, fire doors closed, safe storage of flammable products in compliance with regulations and a programme of checking fire alarms and fire appliances by a nominated person. The potential for fire requires constant consideration and demands appropriate action planning to ensure a safe working environment.

Principles of Safe Practice in The Perioperative Environment

Environment - *Section 1*

LASERS

Introduction

The development of medical lasers has revolutionised surgery. There are many different types of lasers used routinely in the operating department for a wide range of procedures. Since the MDA (Medical Devices Agency) Guidelines on Laser Safety, published in 1995, more sophisticated lasers have been introduced. Each laser should be considered as requiring different operational techniques and will demand consideration of variances in associated hazards. It is therefore essential that the particular manufacturer's instructions and recommendations are adhered to at all times. It is also necessary to consider that the policies and procedures that are developed are in conjunction with the Risk Assessment Guide (NATN 1995).

The following principles will address general aspects related to the safe use of surgical lasers.

What is a laser?

The word LASER is an acronym of the process in which high energy light is created.

LIGHT
AMPLIFICATION (by)
STIMULATED
EMISSION (of)
RADIATION

In this instance, the term radiation applies to light energy only.

Laser light is formed when an electron is a lasting medium (usually gas or crystal) is stimulated to produce particles of light. This stimulation is brought about by the application of energy.

The Properties of Lasers

1. **Collimation**

   Laser light can be thought of as a parallel beam of light which is highly directional. This property, makes lasers very accurate aiming devices. In theory the collimated laser light travels into infinity, demanding safety precautions to prevent accidents and injury.

2. **Coherence**

   Ordinary light travels in random waves, in contrast laser light features waves that are in harmony (in phase). Particles of laser light leave the source and travel in harmonised wave forms arriving at the target tissue at the same moment. This produces a more concentrated form of light than ordinary light.

3. **Monochromatic Light**

   Lasers usually produce light of one colour. Some lasers produce a single green laser light while carbon dioxide lasers produce a single band of infra red light. It is important to remember that laser light is not always visible and care should be taken accordingly. The exception to this rule of monochromic light is the Argon laser which may have up to eleven different colours. In the surgical argon laser there are two bands - blue and green.

BIBLIOGRAPHY

AORN 1997 Laser Safety in the Practice Setting. Standards, Recommended Practices and Guidelines. Denver, AORN Inc.

BSI 1994 Radiation safety of laser products, equipment classification, requirements and user's guide. EN 60825-1. London, BSI

BSI 1993 Medical electrical equipment Part 2 : Particular requirements for the safety of diagnostic therapeutic laser equipment. BS EN 60601-2-22 (IEC 601-2-22: 1922; BS724 : Section 2.122:1993)

BSI 1994 Specification for Filters and Equipment used for personal eye protection against laser systems. BS EN 207

BSI 1995 Guidance on Airway Management during laser surgery of upper airway. ISO TR 11991. London, BSI

BSI 1998 Trachael tubes deisgned for laser surgery. Requirements for marking and accompanying information. ISO 14408. London, BSI

Frost J 1993 Clinical Applications of Lasers. Professional Nurse. 8(5) 298-303

Health and Safety at Work Act 1974 (England, Wales and Scotland)

Health and Safety at Work Order 1978 (Northern Ireland)

Health and Safety at Work Amendments Regulations 1994 (England, Wales and Scotland)

Hill P D 1992 Lasers and Theatre Nursing. British Journal of Theatre Nursing. 1 (10) 18-19

Hill P D 1992 Understanding Lasers. British Journal of Theatre Nursing. 1 (11) 15

Management of Health and Safety at Work Regulations 1992 (England, Wales and Scotland)

Management of Health and Safety at Work Regulations 1993 (Northern Ireland)

MDA 1996 Guidance of the safe use of lasers in Medical and Dental Practice DB9602

MDA 1994 Reporting Adverse Incidents Relating to Medical Devices. SN 9801 (updated each year)

MDA The Re-use of Medical Devices Supplied for Single use only. DB 9501 (updated each year)

NATN 1995 Risk Assessment Guidelines. Harrogate, NATN

Nursing Homes and Nursing Agencies Act 1971 (Northern Ireland)

Nursing Homes and Nursing Agencies Order 1985 (Northern Ireland)

Registered Homes Act 1984 (England and Wales)

Taylor M Campbell C 1998 Lasers In: Clarke P Jones J Surgical Prepraration. Brigdens Operating Department Practice, Edinburgh, Churchill Livingstone

Recommendations for Inclusion in Local Policy

The following issues should be addressed when preparing local laser policies:-

1. Potential Hazards Associated with Lasers
2. General Standard to Protect Patients and Staff
3. Potential Hazards Associated with Lasers

1. Potential Hazards Associated with Lasers

a. Electrical

    i. All laser equipment should adhere to British Safety standard BS EN 60825-1 and where relevant BS EN 60601-2-22.

    ii. Inspection should be carried out by the organisations nominated medical electronics officer, prior to planning and installation.

b. Fire

    All lasers currently used in surgery are thermal lasers which create a very high temperature to vaporise tissue. Adequate precautions are therefore essential to prevent the risk of fire. A carbon dioxide fire extinguisher must be available in theatre at all times and staff must have received training in its use.

i. Anaesthetic gases will support combustion therefore an effective anaesthetic scavenging system must be in place. In addition non-flammable endrotracheal intubation tubes should be used where there is a risk of damage from laser radiation (BSI 1995). Such tubes should be considered mandatory for head and neck surgery.

ii. Non-flammable skin preparation fluids must be used. (Betadine, whilst non inflammable will give off toxic fumes if the laser is fired into a pool of solution).

iii. Particular care must be taken as there is potential risk of setting fire to the surgical drapes, close observation of clinical drapes during the laser procedure is critical.

c. Eye and Skin Injury

i. Laser light can strike the cornea of the eye causing vaporisation and possible destruction to the outer layer, Laser light may also pass through the cornea, be focused by the lens and destroy the retina. When lasers are in use, laser safety eye wear must be worn. Protective eye wear is laser specific as it must be of the appropriate optical density, therefore, it is essential that the correct eye protection is used by staff and patients at all times. Additional protection may be achieved for the unconscious patients by securing the patients eyelids with tape. For head, face and neck surgery further protection may be achieved by using eye pads moistened with saline and protecting the eyes further with goggles. (BS EN 207 and 208).

ii. For laser surgery involving skin, additional protection may be afforded surrounding surface areas, by gauze moistened in saline.

iii. Surgical instruments should have a non-reflective surface and be blackened for visible laser radiation to reduce the potential risk of reflection of the laser beam.

iv. To avoid accidental injury it is essential that clear communication is maintained at all times between the surgeon and the team when lasers are in use. There should therefore be a strict procedure for communicating with the laser operator (surgeon), via the scrub nurse, which must be adhered to at all times.

d. Infective Agents in Laser Plume (smoke)

i. All thermal instruments used in surgery produce smoke. It is possible that infective agents can be present in the laser plume which may be a potential risk to staff.

ii. Dedicated smoke evacuation machines must be used to remove the smoke and the smoke evacuation filters should be checked and changed as per manufacturer's recommendations.

iii. Piped hospital suction apparatus must not be used for smoke evacuation and it is further recommended that portable units are not suitable.

iv. High-filtration surgical masks for laser use should be worn during procedures that produce plume to minimise inhalation of the larger carbonaceous particles.

2. **General Standard to Protect Patients and Staff**

a. Patient safety issues

i. Patients should be afforded appropriate preoperative explanation of laser procedures and precautions, the details of which should be recorded in the patient care plan.

b. Staff safety issues

  i. Any staff member who will be involved in surgical procedures involving a laser must have undertaken a training programme and have been assessed as having the knowledge and skills to participate in the use of the equipment. The individual practitioner must acknowledge their competence to participate and this should be recorded in their personal portfolio/personnel file.

  ii. For each specific laser in an operating department, authorised operators and safety officers must be clearly identified within the local policy. These individuals will carry total responsibility for security of the laser keys and safe practice for that area of care.

  iii. When the laser is in use it is essential to:

      a) restrict access to the laser theatre
      b) reduce the number of people present in that theatre
      c) use warning signs and lights as indications of laser in use
      d) when the laser is in use it is recommended that class 3B and 4 lasers incorporate a remote interlock facility (BS EN 60825-1)

  iv. When not in use the laser must be kept in a secure place. The keys should be kept in a locked cupboard. A register of the laser key issue must be maintained. A laser log book must be updated each time the laser is used with specific records of laser operations, surgical procedure and personnel present in the area of care. This information should also be entered into the patients notes.

  v. All laser incidents/accidents should be recorded on a special incident/accident form and reported to the Unit Laser Safety Officer who in turn will notify the Regional Laser Safety Protection Adviser. In addition, laser incidents must be reported in accordance with local incident/accident policies.

  vi. Occupational health and surveillance in particular opthalmic examination of personnel participating in the use of lasers is recommended (BS EN 60825-1).

c. Obligation of the Employer with regard to the Health and Safety at Work.

  i. The legislation identified in the Health and Safety at Work Act (1974) places a duty on the employers to maintain a working environment for employees that is as safe as is reasonably practicable. This duty extends to incorporate the environment, safe equipment, safe systems of work as well as providing the necessary education, training and supervision to ensure safe working practices.

      A duty of care is also to be extended to ensure the safety of visitors and patients.

  ii. Employees have a duty to consider their own role and contribution in maintaining a safe working environment; employees are required to exercise reasonable care in maintaining safety of the working environment, for themselves and those who may be so affected by their practice, (colleagues, visitors and patients).

  iii. Employees are required to co-operate with the reasonable instructions of their employer to secure and maintain a safe working environment.

Principles of Safe Practice in The Perioperative Environment

Environment - *Section 1*

ELECTRO-SURGICAL EQUIPMENT - DIATHERMY

Introduction

In this section recommendations are set out on the safe use of electrosurgical equipment within the operating department. It is also necessary to consider that the policies and procedures that are developed are in conjunction with the Risk Assessment Guide (NATN 1995).

BIBLIOGRAPHY

Principles of Electrosurgery Safety. 3M UK Plc

AORN 1997 Electrosurgery. Standards, Recommended Practices and Guidelines. Denver, AORN Inc.

Bell A F 1986 Principles and Hazards of Electrocautery in Otolaryngology Otolaryngol. Head and Neck Surgery. 94 (4) 504-507

Butler M Nettheim G 1977 Electrosurgery. Principles and Practice. AORN Journal. 10(3) 21-24

Drew 1980 Quality Assurance of Electrosurgical Devices: A manufacturers view. In: Brigden R J 1988 Electricity and Electromedical Equipment. Operating Theatre Technique 5th Edition. London, Churchill Livingstone

Cobb G V 1996 Tissue Cutting and Coagulation by Computerised Dipolar Electrosurgery. Nuvotek, Leeds

DOH 1990 Ignition of Spirit-Based Skin Cleaning Fluid by Surgical Diathermy Setting Fire to Disposable Surgical Drapes Resulting in Patient Burns. HC (Hazard) (90) 25

Eschmann Limited 1991 Safety Regulations related to Electrosurgical Equipment. Eschmann Bros and Walsh Ltd. Lancing

Evaluation of Surgical Diathermy Units. Journal Med. Eng Technol 1985 November/December 9(6) 281-3

Hoglan M 1995 Potential Hazards from Electrosurgery Plume. Recommendations for Surgical Smoke Evacuation. Canadian Operating Room Nurses Journal 13 (14) 10-16

HSE 1993 Electricity at Work : Safe Working Practices. HS(G) 85

Keymed Radio-Frenquency Cutting and Coagulation in Endoscopic Use. Olympus, Keymed

Levine P A et al 1986 Electrocautery and Pacemakers: Management of the Paced Patient subject to Electrocautery. Ann. Thoracic Surgery. 41(3) 313-317

Leith I M 1980 Electrical Safety in the Hospital. The American Journal of Nursing, 1344-1348

MDA 1996 Risk of Skin Burns from Lead Adapters with Electrosurgical Equipment SN9609

MDA 1996 Xray Equipment : Safety of Footswitches used in adverse conditions SN 9613

MDA 1998 Electrosurgery Accessories such as Monopolar and Bipolar Leads, Footswitches, Handpieces, Graspers and Forceps SN9815 sn 9609

NATN 1995 Risk Assessment Guide (RAG) Harrogate, NATN

NATN 1998 Safeguards for Invasive procedures: the Management of Risks. Harrogate, NATN

Medical Instrumentation No 14 255-256

Valleylab 1996 REM Polyhesive Patient Return Electrodes. Boulder, Valleylab Inc.

Waldran R P 1984 Surgical Diathermy a Potential Hazard. British Journal of Clinical Practice. 38 (7-8) 283

Wainwright D 1988 Diathermy: How safe Is It? British Journal of Theatre Nursing. 25 (1) 7-8

Wicker C P 1991 Working with Electrosurgery. NATN Harrogate

Wicker C P 1992 Making Sense of Electrosurgery. Nursing Times, 88, 45, 31-33

Wicker C P 1993 Principles of Electrosurgery. Scope. Pentax Medical, Harrow

Wicker C P 1996. Working with Electrosurgery (Multimedia Edition). Harrogate, NATN

Wicker C P 1997 Aspects of Safety 1 : Electrosurgery In: Mason J and Shepard M (Eds) 1997 Practical Endoscopy. London, Chapman and Hall

Wicker C P 1998 Principles, Uses and Hazards of Electrosurgery. In: Clarke P Jones J Surgical Preparation. Brigdens Operating Department Practice. Edinburgh, Churchill Livingstone

DHSS 1982 Management of Equipment (January) HEI 98

Health & Safety Executive 1984. Protection Against Electric Shock (Guidance Notes GS27)

Safety Information Bulletin 1982 Severe Burns caused by Chemical Action with Diathermy Plates. (September) 6

Safety Information Bulletin 1985 Loss of Diathermy Plate Monitor Function Due to Defective Dry Place Electrode Holders. (January) 3

Safety Information Bulletin 1987 Surgical Diathermy Avoiding Patient Burns.(September) 66

Safety Information Bulletin 1988 Insulation of Bi-Polar Diathermy Dissecting Forceps. (September) 59

Safety Information Bulletin 1988 Insulation of Bi-Polar Diathermy Avoiding Patient Burns. (September) 66

Royal College of Surgeons of England 1995 Basic Skills for Laparoscopic. Safety Action Bulletin. London

DHSS Guidance

DHSS 1975 Electro-Medical Equipment Hospital Services Engineering Data

DHSS 1982 Evaluation of Surgical Diathermy Units (April) HEI 99

Recommendations for Inclusion in Local Policy

The following issues should be addressed when preparing local policies regarding electrosurgery:-

1. Mono Electrosurgery
2. Bi Polar Electrosurgery
3. New Developments
4. Hazards of Electrosurgery:-
   a. Accidental Burns
   b. Other hazards
5. Preparation of Personnel
6. Maintenance of Equipment
7. Safe Practice
8. Patient Safeguards

1. Monopolar Electrosurgery

A high frequency current is passed through the patient's body from the live electrode (for example, pencil or forceps) to the return electrode (previously called the patient plate or indifferent electrode). The innate resistance of the tissues to the flow of current causes a rise in temperature. The rise in temperature of the tissues is related, in part, to the area of tissue involved and the power of the current. A very small electrode, such as the active electrode, provides sufficient current density to create a high temperature at the point of entry. This high temperature is used to control haemorrhage by coagulation (desiccation or fulguration) or to cut tissues by cell disruption. The current then passes through the body on its way to the return electrode. The relatively large surface area of the return electrode results in a lower current density than is present at the active electrode, so ensuring that the rise in temperature of the tissues at this point is kept to a minimum. The current then returns to the generator.

2. Bipolar Electrosurgery

a. In bipolar electrosurgery the active and return electrodes are combined within the instrument. These electrodes are separated by insulating material. One tine of the forceps is therefore the active electrode, the other tine is the return electrode. Electrosurgery occurs at both tines since they are of similar size.

b. The current passes from one electrode to the other point of contact with the tissues. The pathway is inherently safer than a monopolar pathway as it is much shorter (normally only a few millimetres long) and so the problems associated with alternative pathways are reduced.

c. Bipolar electrosurgery is recommended in situations when:-

   i. Only coagulation is required.

   ii. Coagulation will be required during surgery to peripheral areas of the body, for example, during circumcision.

   iii. Pinpoint or micro coagulation is required, for example, during neurosurgery, ophthalmic surgery or plastic surgery.

   iv. The patient has a pacemaker in situ and the current pathway passes through the heart.

3. New Developments

a. Developments within electrosurgery have intensified as a result of the intense technological research going into minimally invasive surgery. Some recent advances include:-

   i. Active electrode monitoring systems (which can monitor the active electrode for signs of capacitive coupling and insulation failure).

   ii. Instant response generators (which sense the tissue resistance and alter the power of electrosurgical current accordingly).

   iii. Electrosurgical wave manipulation (which has led to reduced power requirements).

   iv. Bipolar cutting tissue.

   v. Monopolar electrosurgery without the need for a return electrode (Dipolar electrosurgery).

b. The high rate of development of new instruments and techniques makes it mandatory practice to ensure that regular updating of education occurs in order to ensure a high level of patient care and safety.

4. Hazards Of Electrosurgery

a. Accidental Burns

   i. This hazard represents the most significant danger to the patient and accounts for around 4% of all negligence claims in the medico-legal arena. The return electrode has been targeted as one of the main problem areas. Although modern generators are isolated and are often equipped with sophisticated monitoring systems, alternative pathways can still arise.

   ii. Alternative pathways occur when the current is diverted from the return electrode and finds an alternative path from the patient to 'ground'. In an isolated generator 'ground' represents the negative phase of the isolation transformer within the electrosurgical generator. In an 'earthed' generator, 'ground' represents the common earth of the mains electricity system. If the point of contact between the patient and the grounded object is small, sufficient current density can be generated to cause a burn. The most likely alternative pathway is created by the patient coming into contact with a metal part of the operating table, a table accessory, or through an ECG electrode. This problem is reduced, but not eliminated, by the use of isolated electrosurgical units which have little or no reference to 'earth'. It is important to realise that, because of the properties of electrosurgical current, earthed referenced currents can still be produced by an isolated generator under certain circumstances.

   iii. Minimally invasive surgery has increased the awareness of direct coupling, capacitive coupling and insulation failure, because of the relatively high numbers of instruments in close proximity within the abdomen at any one time. Any one of these three phenomena may lead to accidental damage to the internal organs of the patient. A knowledge of the principles associated with these phenomena is therefore essential if accidental burning to patients is to be avoided.

b. Other Hazards of Electrosurgery

   i. Interaction with skin disinfection solutions: For example ignition of alcohol based fluids caused by sparks from the active electrode and chemical burns around the site of the return electrode due to pooling and entrapment of fluids.

   ii. Interference with other electromedical devices: This could include pacemakers,

ECG machines and video equipment in minimally invasive surgery.

   iii. Inhalation of the electrosurgical plume.

   iv. Accidental electrocution of the patient or staff with low frequency mains electricity.

5. Preparation of Personnel

a. The greatest defence against accidental patient burns is a well educated staff, therefore constant education and assessment is essential.

b. A regular audit of equipment and procedures should be carried out in order to highlight areas of good practice and to identify areas where improvement in technique or education is necessary.

6. Maintenance of Equipment

a. All cables and electrodes should be checked prior to use in order to ensure that all insulation is intact.

b. The manufacturer's instructions on checking the alarm system should be followed prior to use.

c. Regular planned preventative maintenance checks should be established and a record kept.

7. Safe Practice

a. Ensure all connections are secure prior to commencement of surgery.

b. The active electrode should be housed in an insulated container and kept well away from the operative field during surgery.

c. Electrode gel, if recommended, should be used in accordance with the manufacturer's instructions. Pre-gelled, self adhesive plates are recommended.

d. The activation of the active electrode is the responsibility of the operating surgeon.

e. The electrosurgical generator should be switched off or set to 'standby' before touching the live electrode terminal.

f. Single-use return electrodes should not be re-used.

g. It is the responsibility of the users to ensure that the equipment is suitable for the task.

8. Patient Safeguards

a. It is essential that the return electrode site is free from hair, skin lesions, blemishes or scars, prior to the application of the return electrode.

b. The return electrode should be as close the operative site as is practical.

c. The return electrode should be applied over a vascular, muscular area.

d. The return electrode must be in direct and complete contact with the patient. If the patient is moved during surgery it is necessary to recheck the return electrode site.

e. The return electrode should remain dry during surgery and precautions should be taken to prevent pooling of flammable liquids in any cavity, under the body or on the return electrode itself.

f. The patient should not come in contact with 'grounded' metal objects.

g. Skin condition should be checked before and after application of the return electrode.

Principles of Safe Practice in The Perioperative Environment

TOURNIQUET - FOR LIMB SURGERY

Introduction

A tourniquet is a mechanical device used for the temporary control of the circulation of blood during a surgical procedure. It is essential that all staff are made aware of the potential dangers to the patient and therefore should receive specific instruction prior to use.

It is also necessary to consider that policies and procedures devised in relation to this apparatus are in conjunction with the Risk Assessment Guide (NATN 1995).

BIBLIOGRAPHY

AORN 1997 Use of the Pneumatic Tourniquet. Standards, Recommended Practises and Guidelines. Denver, AORN Inc.

Bollens S Arciero R A 1996. The effect of tourniquet use in anterior ligament reconstruction. American Journal of Sports Medicine 24 (6) 758-764

Graham B et al 1993   Occlusion of arterial flow to the extremities at subsystolic pressures through the use of wide cuffed tourniquet cuffs. Clinical Orthopaedics and Related Research. 286 257-261

Klinken C 1955 The effects of tourniquet time in knee arthroscopy patients receiving intra-articular morphine combined with bupivacaine. The Clinical forum for Nurse Anaesthetists. 6 (1) 37-42

Phillips S Lee A 1991 Tourniquets. British Journal of Theatre Nursing. 1(2) 13-16

Recommendations for Inclusion in Local Policy

The following issues should be addressed when preparing local policies regarding electrosurgery:-

1. Indications for use of a tourniquet.
2. Contra-indications for use.
3. Types of Tourniquet.
4. Care and maintenance.
5. General Safeguards.

1. Indications for use of a tourniquet.

    a. Peripheral joint surgery eg; athroplasty of the knee/elbow, athroscopy of the knee.

    b. Hand surgery eg; tendon or nerve repair, carpal tunnel decompression.

    c. Foot surgery eg; correction of hallus valgus.

    d. Osteotomies.

    e. Internal fixation of fractures of the lower arm/leg.

2. Contra-indications for use

a. Blood disease eg; sickle cell.

b. Localised infection of the limb.

c. Regional infections eg; cellulitis.

d. Vascular disease - peripheral.

e. Severe bone trauma.

3. Types of Tourniquet

Two are mainly used:

a. Leak compensating. Such tourniquets will compensate automatically for any loss of pressure

b. Non leak compensating. Such tourniquets require continuous observation and may require recalibration intraoperatively. This should be done by an appropriate trained member of staff.

Manufacturer's instructions should always be followed on all types of tourniquet.

a. Leak compensating

   i. The pressures usually recommended for this type of tourniquet for safe practice are:

      1) Thigh - double the patient's systolic blood pressure on admission.

      2) Arm 50mm Hg above the patient's systolic blood pressure on admission.

      This pressure may be maintained up to two hours.

   ii. The cuffs are inflated from a compressed air supply, cylinder or pump. The equipment usually consists of a control box, which includes a pressure gauge with an air hose attachment and various sizes of cuffs for upper and lower limbs.

   iii. Tourniquets may be applied to two limbs simultaneously. Prior to use it should be tested and calibrated to check for accuracy. A pressure of 200mm Hg is used for this test.

   iv. It is recommended that the inter-operative maintenance pressures of tourniquets should be recorded in the patient's perioperative record/notes.

b. Non-Leak Compensation

   i. This tourniquet is similar in principle to the former, but is not leak proof, therefore the pressure gauge must be continually observed - safe time two hours.

   ii. The cuffs are inflated from a pressurised cylinder of liquid gas or from a hand pump.

   iii. The average pressure for this type of tourniquet is 250mm Hg for the arm and 500mm Hg for the leg. These measurements are standard for all patients irrespective of the individual patient's systolic blood pressure. Inflation pressure is set before inflating the cuff and there will be an initial fall in pressure. Adequate time should be allowed for this to happen. There is no available test apparatus to check the accuracy of this tourniquet.

   iv. It is recommended that inter-operative maintenance pressures of tourniquets should be recorded in the patient's perioperative record/notes.

4. Care and maintenance

Routine checking of the tourniquet system should be carried out before use and on a planned maintenance programme basis, this should include observations for leaking cuff, worn tubing, loose connections, faulty gauge.

5. General Safeguards

a. It is the responsibility of the surgeon to verify and approve the operating pressure to the tourniquet cuff.

b. Because the function of the tourniquet is to provide a bloodless field it is essential that all connections on the system are secure at all times when in use.

c. In the unlikely event of the tourniquet cuff found to be still inflated some time after surgery eg: recovery - the pressure must not be released until the surgeon has been informed. He/she must decide the correct action to take. A record of the incident should be made.

d. The duration of the tourniquet times must be recorded in the patient's notes/records.

e. To maintain adequate support of the patient's limb and ensure satisfactory exsanguination, it is recommended that two people should always be available when applying the tourniquet.

f. The tourniquet control panel should always be visible throughout the procedure.

g. Care should be taken not to have the cuff sited over bony prominences in order to avoid nerve compression and damage whilst inflated.

h. In order for the limb to be exsanguinated the following methods may be used.

   i. Raising the limb to allow the blood to drain.

   ii. Active exsaguination via a roll cylinder or an Esmarch's bandage.

i. It is recommended that a roll cylinder is used as it is considered safer for the patient, providing a regular/even pressure and a faster process at the commencement of surgery.

j. When applying an Esmarch's bandage the following guidelines apply:-

   i. Each turn of the bandage must overlap by approximately 1 inch and the bandage must be held firmly and under continuous tension in order to squeeze as much blood out of the limb as possible.

   ii. When the limb has been completely wrapped up to the cuff, the cuff is inflated to the required pressure by activating the control box.

   iii. When the surgical procedure involves the leg, the limb should be flexed whilst applying the Esmarch's bandage, then held in flexion until the cuff has been inflated.

k. A record of the time that the tourniquet cuff was inflated must be kept. This should be recorded on the wall board in bold figures. The theatre minute clock should be activated. An audible timing device may be used. It is important that the surgeon is informed when the tourniquet reaches one hour and then every 15 minutes until the operation has been completed.

l. The ultimate responsibility for the application and release of the tourniquet is that of the operating surgeon.

Principles of Safe Practice in The Perioperative Environment

Environment - *Section 1*

ENDOSCOPES

Introduction

This section will provide guidelines for the cleaning and disinfection of endoscopes, fibreoptic cables, video attachments and all accessories.

It is necessary to consider that policies and procedures devised in relation to the cleaning and disinfection of such apparatus are in conjunction with Infection Control Policies, COSHH and with the Risk Assessment Guide (NATN 1995).

It must be stressed that the manufacturer's instructions for the care of specific instruments and endoscopes must be followed at all times.

Cleaning and disinfection of the endoscopic equipment is a specialist procedure and should be carried out by staff who have been trained in this area of work. If equipment is not properly cleaned or maintained it becomes an infection risk. In addition, extreme care is required during cleaning to avoid any damage to this expensive equipment. It is essential that staff have a good working knowledge of the relevant equipment.

BIBLIOGRAPHY

AORN 1997 Edoscopes, Use and care of. Standards, Recommended Practices and Guidelines. Denver, AORN Inc.

Babb J R Bradley C R 1995. Endoscope decontamination :where do we go from here. Journal of Hospital Infection. 30, 543-551

Babb J Bradley C R 1995 A review of Gluteraldehyde alternatives. British Journal of Theatre Nursing. 5 (7) 20-24

Bullard J 1991 Use and Abuse of Gluteraldehyde. Nursing Times. 87(38) 70-71

Control of Substances Hazardous to Health Regulations 1988 (Northern Ireland)

Control of Substances Hazardous to Health Regulations 1994 (England, Wales and Scotland)

Control of Substances Hazardous to Health Amendment Regulations 1992 (Northern Ireland)

DOH 1992 Gluteraldehyde Disinfectants : Use and Management. Safety Action Bulletin No 81. London, DOH

East J 1992 Implementing the COSHH Regulations. Nursing Standard. 6 (10) 33-35

EH 65/32. Gluteraldehyde Criteria Document. HSE Books

Endoscopy Committee Working Party of the BSG 1988 Cleaning and disinfection of equipment for gastrointestinal flexible endoscopy : interim report in GUT. 29 (8) 1134-1151

Endoscopy Committee Working Party of the 1993 BSG Aldehyde Disinfectants and Health in Endoscopy Units in GUT. 34: 1641-1645

Health and Safety at Work Act 1974

NHS Estates 1994 Health Building Note 52 volume 2 Accommodation for day care endoscopy unit. HMSO

HSE 1997 Gluteraldehyde CHAN 7. September

HSE 1998 Gluteraldehyde and You. Information Leaflet. Autumn

Hutson P Dodd M 1993 A cause for concern. British Journal of Theatre Nursing. 2 (10) 10-12

Hutt G 1994 Gluteraldehyde Revisited. British Journal of Theatre Nursing. 3 (10) 10-11

Menzies D 1995 Gluteraldehyde : Controlling the risk to health. British Journal of Theatre Nursing. 4 (11) 13-15

NATN 1995 Risk Assessment Guide (RAG). Harrogate, NATN

NATN 1998 Infection Control. Principles of Safe Practice in the Perioperative Environment. Harrogate, NATN

NATN 1998 Universal Precautions. Principles of Safe Practice in the Perioperative Environment. Harrogate, NATN

Wicks J 1994 Handle with Care. Nursing Times. 90 (13) 67-70

Recommendations for Inclusion in Local Policy

It should be remembered that patients undergoing endoscopic procedures require the same support and considerations whether they are under sedation or anaesthesia.

All patients undergoing endoscopic procedures must be considered 'at risk' and consistent with 'Universal precautions', appropriate measures should be taken to reduce incidence of cross-infection with HIV, Hepatitis B and other Microorganisms

The following issues should be addressed when preparing local policies regarding endoscopes:-

1. General Disinfectant Guidance
2. Protection of Staff

1. General Disinfectant Guidance

a. Endoscopy is considered to be an invasive procedure and as such, all precautions should be taken to protect staff and patients from cross infection, whatever the micro-organism.

b. Thorough cleaning of the instrument is vital. Cleaning failure will result in inadequate disinfection and sterilisation of the equipment. During cleaning, the equipment should be inspected for any damage or malfunction.

c. Flexible scopes should be cleaned and disinfected in enclosed automated washers.

d. i. The preparation and use of disinfection solutions must be carried out according to the manufacturer's recommendations and these should be strictly adhered to at all times.

ii. The time that the endoscopes are in contact with the disinfectants should be stated specifically. This time period can be determined with the Infection Control Specialist as per local policy and contact times before, between and after the list must be specifically stated.

iii. A clock timer should be used for accuracy and if an automatic or semi automatic cleaner/disinfector is not available.

iv. Exhaust, ventilation and fume cabinets must be in place to reduce the exposure of staff have to the fumes from the disinfectant agent, thus reducing the risk of allergic reaction.

v. Liaison with the Occupational Health Department is advised to ensure a system of health surveillance is in place.

e. It is essential that staff adhere to the cleaning procedures. Clear guidelines for the use of disinfectant and the protection of staff should be displayed at all times in the preparation and/or cleaning areas.

f. Aldehyde based solutions should be disposed of through a closed disposal system (eg: plumbed in washers) that minimises the risk of staff exposure.

g. The DOH recommends the use of steam for sterilisation as a method of choice wherever possible, according to the manufacturer's guidelines eg: rigid scopes.

h. i. All endoscopes should be decontaminated and dried thoroughly before storage. All moving parts should be lubricated according to manufacturer's instructions.

ii. During storage it is essential that flexible endoscopic equipment is supported on specifically designed wall brackets, to ensure that drying is effective and that the equipment is protected from damage.

iii. A well ventilated lockable cupboard is recommended for storage as the cost implication of accidental damage is high.

i. A certificate of decontamination is required for any equipment sent for repair or returned from loan.

j. It is recommended that a planned preventative maintenance programme is in place for endoscopic equipment.

2. Protection of Staff

Staff working in the endoscopy room/theatre are at risk from infection transmitted from the patient and also from sensitivity to disinfectants in use. All staff should be offered protection against Hepatitis virus by vaccination and their anti-body status checked following immunisation.

a. Safeguards against infection

i. Open cuts, fresh abrasions and other skin lesions in patients and staff should be covered with a waterproof dressing.

ii. Endoscopy staff should wear disposable waterproof aprons to avoid splashes on clothing. Goggles or glasses must be worn as eye splashes with blood or solution are likely. Eyewash bottles should be readily available. Disposable gloves of a density to afford adequate protection should be worn throughout the procedure.

b. Accidental Injury

i. Special care must be taken with the handling of sharp instruments and needles as gloves provide no protection against inoculation injury.

ii. Routine barrier precautions should be observed when in contact with blood or body fluids.

c. Safeguards against sensitivity to Aldehydes

i. Alternative methods of sterilisation and disinfection should be investigated

e.g.: non-aldehyde based chemicals use of autoclavable rigid scopes

ii. Sensitivity arises from splashing (which can affect the eyes) from hand immersions and from inhalation of vapour. Reactions may include dermatitis, conjunctivitis, nasal irritation and asthma. Both employers and employees are reminded of their dual responsibility in complying with Health and Safety At Work Act (1974) and COSHH, in the promotion of staff health.

Principles of Safe Practice in The Perioperative Environment

Environment - *Section 1*

INFECTION CONTROL

Introduction

The environmental design and architectural layout of operating departments have developed and improved in order to minimise the risks of hospital acquired infections and to promote optimum infection control.

The greatest source of micro-organisms is people and the design of the operating theatre complex alone, will not compensate for poor practice. Therefore it is essential that high standards of practice are adhered to at all times by **all** members of the multi-disciplinary team.

It is necessary to consider that policies and procedures devised in relation to infection control are in conjunction with the Risk Assessment Guide (NATN 1995).

All theatre personnel have an individual responsibility to ensure that all practices within their operating departments are evidence based and adhered to. The evidence base informing practice should be reviewed and updated at agreed intervals and on **not less** than one occasion per year.

The aim of infection control is to prevent infection, cross infection and auto infection through human and inanimate contact.

These principles do not stand in isolation but should be read in conjunction with the recommendations set out in Clinical Practice, Preparation of Personnel, Visitors to the Perioperative Environment, Scrubbing, Gowning and Gloving, Aspetic Techniques.

BIBLIOGRAPHY

AORN 1997 Environmental Cleaning in the Practice Setting. Standards, Recommended Practices and Guidelines for Perioperative Nursing. Denver, AORN Inc.

NHS Estates 1991 Health Building Note 26 Operating Department. HMSO

NHS Estates 1993 A Strategic guide to clinical waste management. (EEL(94)1)

DOH 1994 Clinical Waste Management. HSG (94) 50

DOH 1995 Disposal of Clinical Waste. (EPL(95)33)

Health & Safety at Work Act 1974

Howell G 1998 Something in the Air. British Journal of Theatre Nursing. 8 (1) 29-32

HSE 1996 RIDDOR '96

NATN 1995 Risk Assessment Guide (RAG). NATN Harrogate

NATN 1998 Preparation of Personnel. Principles of Safe Practice in the Perioperative Environment. NATN Harrogate

NATN 1998 Scrubbing, Gowning and Gloving. Principles of Safe Practice in the Perioperative Environment. NATN Harrogate

NATN 1998 Visitors in the Perioperative Environment. Principles of Safe Practice in the Perioperative Environment. NATN Harrogate

NATN 1998 Aseptic Techniques. Principles of Safe Practice in the Perioperative Environment. NATN Harrogate

NHS Estates 1994 Ventilation in healthcare premises. HTM 2025

NHS Estates 1994 Clinical waste incineration joint venture. HGN ISBN 0013217684

NHS Estates 1995 Safe disposal of clinical waste - whole hospital policy guidance. HGN ISBN 0113221967

Recommendations for Inclusion in Local Policy

A policy for control of infection should be developed in collaboration or agreement with the local Infection Control Officer. Four distinct areas should be considered, these are:-

1. Preparation of Personnel
2. Preparation and Maintenance of Equipment/Environment
3. Preparation and storage of sterile instruments
4. Patient safeguards

1. Preparation of Personnel

To be read in conjunction with Preparation of Personnel within this document. The following principles apply to all staff working within the perioperative environment.

   a. Health

   i. Within an operating department environment it is important that all staff are in an optimum state of health and any incidents of ill health eg: skin lesion or sore throats must be reported to the team leader who will advise on appropriate action.

   ii. It is mandatory that all personnel receive the Hepatitis B vaccine.

   iii. All personal injuries or ill health occurring at work, must be reported to the manager and statutory and local procedures followed (RIDDOR 1996). The theatre manager should liaise and take advice from the Occupational Health Officer and Infection Control Co-ordinator.

   iv. Under the Health and Safety at Work Act 1974 all individuals should take responsibility for ensuring their own health and safety and should report/seek advice regarding concerns or hazardous practices to the local Health and Safety Officer.

   b. Personal Hygiene

   All operating departments should have established principles and standard statements which outline the standards of personal hygiene required by all members of staff within the perioperative environment. Hygiene standards should be viewed as a matter of personal responsibility.

   c. Clothing/Footwear

   As theatre clothing and footwear is an integral part of infection control the operating department should have locally approved principles and standard statements regarding theatre clothing and footwear. Standards should be adhered to when entering and leaving all areas of the operating department.

2. Preparation and Maintenance of Equipment/Environment

   a. Planned preventative maintenance programmes are an essential part of preventing infection by ensuring that:

   i. All medical and electrical equipment is examined for potential faults and cleaned in accordance with manufacturer's instructions and local guidelines.

   ii. All medical and electrical equipment requiring repair/servicing or for loan requires a decontamination certificate before leaving the department.

   iii. Records relating to maintenance and cleaning of equipment and environment must be maintained.

   b. Ventilation, Temperature and Humidity of the Environment

   i. The environment should be safe, comfortable and organised.

ii. Temperature and humidity must be checked daily, and recorded as recommended. Optimum temperature and humidity settings minimise microbial growth.

iii. Ventilations should occur via total loss system which prevents re-circulation of air (NHS Estates 1994). There should be a total air exchange of 20 cycles per minute in the immediate theatre area. Air changes required in adjacent rooms (eg. recovery and ancillary rooms) will be less than this and will be governed by the transfer grill design.

iv. Positive pressure ventilation provides the rapid removal of contaminants and therefore there should be no unnecessary opening or closing of doors.

v. All mechanical and engineering systems (ventilation, temperature and humidity systems) within a theatre complex should be subject to regular maintenance according to the manufacturer's recommendations. Clear documentation and records should be maintained.

vi. The use of settle plates for bacteriological assessment following commissioning of a theatre or 'high' cleaning should be governed by local policy or on the recommendation of the Infection Control Officer.

c. Domestic Cleaning

i. Domestic cleaning of all equipment, furniture and surfaces must be of a high standard ensuring cleansing is in accordance with manufacturers' instructions and local infection control policies.

ii. All cleaning fluids must be used in accordance with manufacturing instructions and local infection control policies.

iii. Disposal of contaminated waste material should be in accordance with national and local policies.

iv. The cleaning of an operating department should be monitored by a designated responsible person; monitoring should include a review of cleaning schedules (eg: aspects of cleaning and frequency). Records should be maintained.

3. **Preparation and storage of sterile instruments**

a. There should be a designated separate store for sterile equipment and instruments.

b. Aseptic preparation of equipment and instruments should be carried out in a designated room with appropriate and recommended ventilation.

c. Procedures for cleansing, disinfection and sterilisation must be strictly observed and carried out following manufacturer's and local infection control guidelines.

4. **Patient Safeguards**

a. Liaison with ward staff is essential to ensure that the preparation of the patient for surgery is at optimum level and in accordance with locally agreed policies.

b. When the patient is transferred to the operating department on a bed or trolley it is important to adhere to local policy for transferring patients to avoid infection risks. Local policies should address issues such as change of bed linen and cleansing of trolley/bed frames.

c. The commonest source of wound infection is the patient's own skin, therefore the principles of skin preparation are designed to reduce bacterial flora of the skin. In the instance of known allergic sensitivity, a selection of skin preparations are available to suit all individual needs. Effectiveness of skin preparation is related to the efficiency of skin preparation which is directly related to the efficiency of application. Evidence based guidance on the appropriate selection and application of skin preparations, should form the basis for local policy.

d. Surgical drapes provide another important barrier against infection. The efficient and correct use of these is related to the fabric and method of draping. Drapes should be impervious, fluid repellent and form a barrier between the patient and external environment.

e. **Aseptic technique is essential for infection control. All staff must apply and maintain this principle at all times.**

f. On completion of the operative procedure careful consideration should be given to:

    i.   Whether a wound requires a surgical dressing.

    ii. The choice of dressing required.

    iii. The reason for the dressing.

g. Infection control must be maintained throughout the postoperative phase and patients must be nursed on a clean, warm and dry bed or trolley.

h. All wounds drains and catheters provide an ideal entry site for bacterial contamination and therefore the principles of aseptic technique and wound care should apply.

Principles of Safe Practice in The Perioperative Environment

Environment - *Section 1*

RADIATION PROTECTION

Introduction

Ionising radiation is used widely in all operating departments. Recent developments in radiology have facilitated non-invasive surgical procedures in many specialities. This increase in the number of intraoperative X-rays has raised the potential risk to perioperative staff.

Technological refinements have improved the safety aspects of radiation equipment. In general, most staff are exposed to very low radiation doses. Theatre staff must however be aware that this medium carries a risk and it is essential that staff adhere to the national radiation regulations and policy at all times. Each organisation of the United Kingdom (England, Ireland, Scotland and Wales) has its own particular publication, which itemises the nationally approved Codes of Practice.

Each organisation will have an appointed Radiation Protection Adviser who must be consulted when a local policy is developed. This principle will offer specialist safeguards for inclusion in a local operating department policy. Each hospital should appoint a local Radiation Protection Officer to take responsibility within the Operating Department.

BIBLIOGRAPHY

HSE 1985 The Ionising Radiation Regulations SI 1985 No 1333 London

The Ionising Radiation Regulations (Northern Ireland) 1985 Belfast

HSE 1985 Guidance Notes for the Protection of Persons Against Ionising Radiation Arising from Medical and Dental Use: Joint Body Recommendations

Health and Safety Agency 1985 The Ionising Radiation Regulations (Northern Ireland) Protection of Persons Against Ionising Radiation Arising from any Work Activity: Approved Code of Practice HMSO Belfast

Lewis C 1994 Radiation Protection. Nursing Standard. 8 (22) 54

NATN 1998 Potential Hazards to Staff. Principles of Safe Practice in the Perioperative Environment. Harrogate, NATN

Wicker T 1994 Radiation Safety in the Operating Department. British Journal of Theatre Nursing. 4 (6) 20

Recommendations for Inclusion in Local Policy

The following issues should be addressed when preparing ionising radiation policies:-

1. Use of radiation as a method of diagnosis and an aid to surgery
2. Use of radio-active sources as a method of treatment eg: caesium implants.

1. Use of radiation as a method of diagnosis and an aid to surgery, general recommendations:

a. All staff have a responsibility to protect themselves and others. They should not knowingly expose themselves or others to radiation more than is necessary. It is essential that staff do not stand in the direct primary beam and a desired distance is maintained from the beam, consistent with relevant duties.

b. Radiation monitoring should be carried out considering the following:

   i. Any incident which may have resulted in unforeseen exposure must be reported immediately to the Radiation Protection Officer for investigation. A record of persons involved must be documented and the incident outlined.

   ii. Any defect identified in monitoring equipment must be reported to the Radiation Protection Officer. The equipment must be taken out of circulation and labelled as defective and only returned to circulation following the recommissioning process.

   iii. Staff working routinely in controlled areas **may** be issued with **personal dosemeters** on the advice of the Radiation Protection Officer.

   iv. A single film badge is used to measure the whole body dose and should be worn on the trunk, at the chest or waist level and under any protective clothing that may be worn.

   v. Where dosemeters are used they should be monitored monthly and documented.

   vi. The results of personal monitoring should be kept at local level by the Radiation Protection Officer and may be inspected by any individual worker before the results are forwarded to the Radiation Protection Adviser.

c. The radiation dose to patients should be kept as low as reasonably practicable whilst maintaining the required dosage to provide diagnostic information. All exposures should be in accordance with accepted practices and additional protection should be considered eg: thyroid, gonodal and ovarian shielding.

d. Only authorised personnel who are trained and assessed may use X-ray equipment. It is their responsibility to ensure a safe environment for all patients and staff present.

   i. Any faults identified in the X-ray equipment or safety systems must be documented and reported to the Radiation Protection Officer.

   ii. Following commissioning all radiation equipment must be subjected to a planned preventative work programme for which clear documentation is maintained.

e. Protective clothing eg: lead aprons and gloves

   i. Each protective garment must be uniquely identified with a code in order that faulty equipment may be withdrawn from use.

ii. Protective garments should be safeguarded from damage and cleaned after use. They should be examined visually at frequent intervals to ensure they remain undamaged. Storage facilities must be available which allow lead aprons to hang freely and singly on appropriate racking.

iii. The Radiation Protection Officer should arrange tests of each protective garment not less than once each year and maintain records accordingly.

iv. Staff who are required to physically support a patient having radiological investigation must wear specialised protective clothing, for example lead gloves. Discretion is required in assessing the degree of risk to staff when maintaining patient safety and providing support.

v. Protective garments should be available and used for patients to prevent undue exposure to harmful rays.

f. Staff who become pregnant must inform their head of department as soon as it is know and seek advice from the Radiation Protection Officer concerning radiation exposure in controlled areas.

g. When X-ray is in use, there is an absolute need to:-

i. Ensure that there are notices displayed to inform people that X-ray equipment is in use, thus restricting access to the area.

ii. Ensure that the theatre team is aware that X-ray procedures are required in order that all relevant equipment is available eg: X-ray tables and protective clothing

iii. Actively promote asepsis when equipment is used in close proximity to

the surgical wound eg: use of sterile covers on equipment.

iv. Maintain a safe environment at all times.

v. Offer a clear explanation to the patient to identify the allergy status of any patient who may undergo an X-ray investigation where a radio-opaque contrast will be used. Iodine allergy is potentially life threatening in this situation and resuscitation equipment must be available.

2. **Use of radioactive sources as a method of treatment, general recommendations:**

a. Operating department staff involved in caring for patients who are undergoing treatment using radioactive sources must receive training in these specialist practices and be assessed accordingly.

b. A local policy must be in place which identifies the designated individuals with responsibility for safe practice. It is essential to ensure that advice regarding particular incidents is forthcoming immediately eg: decontamination procedures.

i. Contact telephone numbers of key staff are essential.

ii. It is strongly recommended that surgery involving radio-active sources is only undertaken when the designated operating department's Radiation Protection Officer is available.

c. Contingency plans should be in place for the following incidences which may occur when radio-active sources are in use:-

i. A patient dies in theatre.

ii. An outbreak of fire.

iii. A loss, a suspected loss or damage to sources.

d. Since active iridium and gold treatments are infrequently used in theatre, it is recommended that a physicist is present to supervise their use.

e. During surgery

   i. When unsealed radioactive sources are used in surgery, it is recommended that two pairs of surgical gloves be worn to give some protection to the hands.

   ii. If surgical gloves are torn and injury occurs to the hands of the scrubbed person the injury should be irrigated immediately with tap water, taking care not to wash the contamination into the wound or spread contamination to other areas of the body. The incident should be recorded and the unit's Radiation Protection Officer contacted immediately.

f. In recovery, where patients are receiving treatment with active implants, their beds should be placed at a minimum of two meters away from occupied beds, alternatively the patient may be isolated in a partitioned area away from other patients.

   i. A notice should be displayed which informs personnel that the patient is receiving treatment with radioactive implants.

   ii. Depending on the radioactivity of implants used, no one nurse should stay with the patient more that 30 minutes.

   iii. Staff should seek advice from the Regional Protection Adviser when planning and implementing care of such patients.

g. At the end of the operation, staff, equipment (which includes the operating tables and instruments etc.) the theatre and recovery room should be monitored for radioactivity.

Principles of Safe Practice in
The Perioperative Environment

Patient Care - *Section 2*

Reviewers

June Champion RGN BA (Hons) Public Policy and Management
Theatre Sister Ophthalmology and Otoloaryngology
Royal Group of Hospitals Trust,
Belfast

Patricia O'Callaghan RGN RSCN
NVQ Co-ordinator
Royal Group of Hospitals Trust
Belfast

Nikki Henning RGN Diploma in Advanced Health Studies
Staff Nurse
Cardiac Theatres
Royal Group of Hospitals Trust
Belfast

Principles of Safe Practice in The Perioperative Environment

Patient Care- *Section 2*

SURGICAL PREPARATION OF THE PATIENT FOR SURGERY

Introduction

The preparation of the patient for surgery within the operating theatre is normally undertaken by the clinician. In certain circumstances it may be delegated to personnel trained to fulfil the role.

Surgical preparation requires knowledge of infection control principles and diligent application of aseptic techniques. It is essential that all grades of staff receive support in these techniques until proficient.

BIBLIOGRAPHY

AORN 1995 Proposed recommended practices for use and selection of barrier materials for surgical gowns and drapes. AORN Journal. 62 (3) 449, 451-453

AORN 1997 Recommended Practices for Perioperative Nursing Standards Recommended Practice Guidelines 3. Denver, AORN Inc.

AORN 1997 Maintaining a sterile field. Standard, Recommended Practices and Guidelines. Denver, AORN Inc.

Belkin N L 1996 More on squaring off ...elimination of squaring off with towels. AORN Journal. 64 (5) 685 - 686

Blacklock B J 1996 Over-draping: a practice question. Canadian Operating Room Journal. 14 (3) 9-11

Consumer Protection Act 1987

Coyne M A 1996 Squaring off .... with cloth towels. AORN Journal. 64 (1) 21

Data Protection Act 1984

DHSS 1987 Hospital laundry arrangement for infected linen HC (87) 30

Dodds F 1996 Under Pressure. British Journal of Theatre Nursing. 6 (9) 33-35

Flanagan M Fletcher J Hollingworth H 1994 Preoperative shaving. Journal of Wound Care. 3 (7) 338

Guide to Good Manufacturing Practices BS 5750 1981

Guide to Good Pharmaceutical Manufacturing Practice 1983

Hallstrom R Beck S L K 1993 Implementations of the AORN Skin Shaving Standard. AORN Journal. 58 (3) 498-506

HSE 1992 Safe Disposal of Clinical Waste.

Jepsen O Bruttomesso K A 1993 The Effectiveness of Perioperative Skin Preparations. AORN Journal. 58 (3) 477-484

NATN 1993 The role of the Nurse as First Assistant in the Operating Department. Harrogate, NATN

NATN 1994 The Nurse as Surgeons Assistant. Harrogate, NATN

NATN 1998 Diathermy. Principles Of Safe Practice In The Perioperative Environment. Harrogate, NATN

NATN 1998 Infection Control. Principles of Safe Practice in the Perioperative Environment. Harrogate, NATN

NATN 1998 Aseptic Technique. Principles of Safe Practice in the Perioperative Environment. Harrogate, NATN

NHS Estates 1994 A Strategic Guide to Clinical Waste Management.

Small S P 1996 Preoperative hair removal : a case report with implications for nursing. Journal of Clinical Nursing. 5 (2) 79-84

UKCC 1992 The Code of Conduct. 3rd Edition. London, UKCC

UKCC 1992 Scope of Professional Practice. London, UKCC

Recommendations for Inclusion in Local Policy

The following issues should be addressed when preparing local policies for surgical preparation of the patient for surgery.

1. Preparation of Patients
2. Equipment and Procedure
3. Draping the Patient

1. Preparation of Patients

Patients should arrive for routine surgery with clear skin, thus reducing the risk of auto - and cross - infection.

a. Prior to preparing the Surgical area, the following must be checked:

  i. The identity of the patient.

  ii. The site of the operation.

  iii. Any allergies noted on the patient's care plan.

  iv. Visual inspection of wounds.

  v. Visual inspection and pressure area assessment using appropriate risk assessment tool.

  vi. The site of the diathermy return electrode plate.

  vii. That the patient is in the required position to facilitate surgery.

b. Routine preoperative hair removal should be avoided if possible. If it is necessary then it should be done with a surgical clipper and disposable blade assembly or a depilatory cream may be used. The procedure must be carried out as close to the time of surgery as possible.

c. The surgical preparation should not commence until all non-sterile personnel who are not members of the surgical team are clear of the operative field.

2. Equipment and Procedure

a. All lotions should be prepared for use in order to comply with the guide for Good Pharmaceutical Manufacturing Practice.

b. In order to comply with the Consumer Protection Act it is necessary to record the expiry date, batch number and supplier of all lotions used.

c. Aqueous based solutions are recommended for skin preparation.

d. Preparation swabs should be positioned on the holder in such a way that the end of the holder cannot traumatise the patient.

e. Only sufficient antiseptic solution should be applied. Great care should be taken to avoid solution running onto the diathermy return electrode plate or pooling under the patient. Care is also required to prevent seepage occurring under tourniquet cuffs.

f. Cleansing should begin at the site of the incision and continued outward in either a rectangle or spiral motion. It is recommended that the swab should not be brought back to the incision site as this would return micro-organisms to the area.

g. An adequate area of skin surface should be prepared in order to allow a safe extension of the incision to be made if this should prove necessary during a surgical procedure.

3. Draping the Patient

a. It is recommended that the patient's skin is dry prior to commencement of the draping procedure.

b. In order to prevent contamination during the draping procedure, scrubbed personnel should ensure that:

   i.   The drapes are intact.

   ii. The drapes are unfolded carefully to waist height.

   iii. The hands are protected by folding the drape around the hand.

   iv. The distal edges of the drapes are allowed to fall naturally.

c. When the sterility of a draping procedure has been compromised complete re-draping should be recommended.

d. It is recommended that non adhesive drapes are held in place by an atraumatic towel clip, to hold the drapes together.

Where adhesive drapes are used, checks should be made of patient's sensitivity to adhesives.

e. Prior to the start of surgery it is recommended that the scrub team check the effectiveness of their draping procedures, paying particular attention to table fitments, etc.

f. The drapes should remain in place until the dressing had been applied.

g. The scrub nurse should be considered the person of choice to dispose of all drapes into the appropriate bags while she is still gowned and gloved.

Principles of Safe Practice in The Perioperative Environment

Patient Care- *Section 2*

SAFE HANDLING AND POSITIONING OF PATIENTS

Introduction

Positioning is a potentially hazardous procedure to both patients and staff. No member of the perioperative team, regardless of their designation, should be allowed to take part unsupervised in the positioning of patients until they have received instruction, and have been assessed as proficient in the techniques involved.

The anticipation of patient's needs and subsequent planning will ensure safe and secure positioning with optimal comfort for the patient. Co-ordinated, successful and competent positioning will afford:-

1. Maximum safety
2. Adequate exposure of the operating site
3. Prevention of unnecessary postoperative complications

The patient's dignity must be observed throughout.

BIBLIOGRAPHY

RCN - A Guide to the Manual Handling of Patients 4th Edition. London, RCN

Health & Safety at Work Act 1994

European Economic Community 1990. Council Directorate on minimum handling of loads. Official Journal of the European Community. No L156/9

HSC 1991 Manual Handling of Loads. Proposals for Regulations and Guidance. London, HSC

Berry & Johns 1992 Operating Room Technique. (7th Edition) Mosby Year Book, USA

Biddle C Cannaby M J 1990 Surgical Positions. AORN Journal. 52 (2) 350-359

Bridel J 1992 Pressure sores and intraoperative risk. Nursing Standard. 7 (21) 28-30

Graling P R Colvin D B 1992 The Lithotomy position in colon surgery AORN Journal. 55 (4) 1029-1035

Green S 1996 Positioning of Patient for Surgery. British Journal of Theatre Nursing. 6 (5) 35-38

Insinger J Bailes B K 1993 Care of the patient undergoing spinal surgery. AORN Journal. 58 (3) 509-519

MacKenzie M Richardson B Kidd R Tracy M 1997 A Novel Limb-Support System to Reduce Postural Load in Theatres. British Journal of Theatre Nursing. 6 (10) 28-30

Walsh J 1993 Postoperative effects of OR positioning. RN. 56 (2) 50-57

Recommendations for Inclusion in Local Policy

Risk Assessment for all positioning should be undertaken and understood by all members of the multidisciplinary team. The four main areas for consideration are:-

1. Assessment of individual patient needs
2. Patient safeguards
3. Specific considerations for individual positions
4. Equipment and safeguards

1. Assessment of Individual Patient Needs

a. The clinical history of each patient should be known before any positioning takes place, thus allowing individual consideration to be given to:-

   i. The physical condition of the patient.

   ii. The nature of surgical intervention.

   iii. Specific individual needs (it may be necessary to seek specialist help at this stage from eg: the physiotherapy department).

b. When positioning patients with physical abnormalities careful consideration is required. For example, no patient should have his or her limbs forced into position, rather a compromise position should be sought.

c. It is essential that sufficient members of staff are made available to ensure the safe positioning of individual patients.

2. Patient Safeguards

a. It is recommended that patients are anaesthetised prior to positioning to facilitate airway management. Anaesthetised patients must only be moved with the anaesthetists' permission.

b. Care must be taken at all times during the positioning procedure to avoid:-

   i. Friction burns.

   ii. Damage to soft tissue eg: genitals of males and breasts of females.

   iii. Damage to eyes from introcular pressure and corneal abrasions.

   iv. Pressure on ears.

   v. Nerve damage.

c. The patient must be carefully positioned over the operating table breaks prior to adjustment of the table.

d. The patient must be prevented from coming into contact with any metal part of the operating table in order to reduce the risk of diathermy burns.

e. Correct and appropriate padding must be used to protect the patient's veins, nerves and bony prominences from pressure.

f. Patient's limbs, joints and spinal lordoses must be supported with appropriate equipment in order to reduce the risk of postoperative pain.

g. At all times the patient's anatomical position must be maintained in order to prevent injury from hyperextension of joints.

h. Preventative measures must be taken to reduce the risk of venostasis.

i. Members of the scrub team must avoid leaning against the patient's body/limbs at all times in order to prevent injury to the patient.

j. Following surgery the condition of the patient's skin should be checked, and any changes in condition documented and action taken as required.

3. Specific considerations for Individual Positions

These are in addition to the recommendations under patient safeguards

a. Lithotomy position

    i. The patient's hands should be comfortably protected to avoid injury when the operating table is adjusted.

    ii. At the commencement and at the end of surgery the patient's legs must be moved simultaneously and with care to prevent pelvic injury and sudden hypertension.

b. Prone position

    In order to prevent post operative neck and upper back pain in a patient positioned on a frame, the patient's pelvis should be kept level with the chest and the head in a neutral position.

c. Lateral position

    i. A padded restraint should be placed around the operating table and pelvis to secure the patient.

    ii. Precautions should be taken against heat loss as this is a particular hazard for patients in this position.

    iii. The operating table must be adjusted gradually to allow the anaesthetist to monitor the patients blood pressure throughout the manoeuvre.

4. Equipment and Safeguards

a. The modern operating table is a complex piece of equipment which must be serviced regularly under a planned preventative maintenance programme in order to ensure optimal patient safety during surgical interventions

b. All controls, brakes and accessories on operating tables must be checked daily prior to use, in order to ensure that they, are clean, in good repair and in working order. All accessories must be correctly and appropriately padded to prevent injury to the patient.

c. Table mattresses should be clean and inspected regularly for any damage and conform to British Standard recommendations.

d. Any equipment which is damaged will compromise patient safety and infection control. It must therefore be immediately taken out of use and labelled for repair.

e. Patient positioning devices should be available, choice of appropriate device should take into account cross infection issues.

Principles of Safe Practice in The Perioperative Environment

Patient Care- *Section 2*

CARE OF THE DECEASED

Introduction

There is relatively little information available to nurses regarding care of the deceased patient within the perioperative environment. Each hospital will have developed general protocols in the event of patient death and these should be adhered to. The aim of this section is to outline the general principles concerning care of the deceased patient in the perioperative environment.

Advances in surgery and anaesthetic techniques have reduced the incidence of unexpected patient death in this environment. Whenever a patient dies suddenly in the perioperative environment there is a legal requirement to establish the cause of death through a post-mortem examination. With the development of transplant surgery however, theatre staff are caring for deceased patients following organ retrieval. For all patients the general principles of care will apply.

BIBLIOGRAPHY

Attwood C 1995 Dying with dignity. Technic. Issue 138, 15

Ayrton N A 1982 Last offices in cases of notifiable disease: the use of cadaver bags in controlling infection. Nursing Times. 12-18

Bender M 1990 The Quality of Dying - how to provide good care of the ill and dying patient. Winslow Press

Chiarella M 1994 Dying with dignity: Recent Developments. ACORN Journal. 7 (1) 17-18

Descheneaux K 1991 Death investigations: how you can help. Nursing 21 (9): 52-55

Edwards J 1997 Sudden Death and the Theatre Nurse. British Journal of Theatre Nursing. 6 (12) 11-14

Green J 1992 Death with Dignity - Christianity. Nursing Times. 88 (3) 26-29

Green J 1992 Death with Dignity - Jehovah's Witness. Nursing Times. 88 (5)

Green J 1992 Death with Dignity - The Mormon Church. Nursing Times. 88 (6) 44-45

Home Office 1971 Report of the Committee on the Death Certification and Coroners. Cmnd 4810

Hutchings D 1991 Spirituality in the face of Death. The Canadian Nurse. 87 (5) 30-31

Jefferies B 1993 Death in the operating room. ACORN Journal. 6 (2) 15-18

NATN 1998 Infection Control. Principles of Safe Practice in the Perioperative Environment. Harrogate, NATN

NATN 1998 Managerial Issues. Principles of Safe Practice in the Perioperative Environment. Harrogate, NATN

Neuberger J 1994. Caring for dying of people of different faith. 2nd Ed Mosby

RCN 1981 Verification of Death and the performances of Last Offices. London, RCN

Speck P 1992 Care after death ... cleansing and shrouding the body. Nursing Times. 88 (6) 2-11

Recommendations for Inclusion in Local Policy

General Considerations

1. If death occurs within the perioperative environment the person in charge must ensure the following personnel are informed immediately, in order to comply with legal requirements.

    a. Operating Department Manager

    b. The ward and/or intensive care staff

It is the responsibility of the medical staff to inform their Senior Colleagues.

2. Local guidelines must include the method of communication in order to ensure that relatives are informed at the earliest opportunity.

3. The requirement of differing faiths and religions must be taken into consideration.

4. If a death occurs within the perioperative environment:

    a. all drains must be left in position

    b. catheters or cannulae should be closed with a spigot

    c. any endotracheal or tracheostomy tubes may be removed

    d. wounds should be covered by a dressing

    e. a cadaver bag should be used

These guidelines may vary locally according to the requirements of the coroner.

5. The care of the deceased patient should be undertaken according to local policy. Trained staff from the patient's previous area of care may be involved in certain situations, for example, unexpected death.

6. Staff should ensure that all documents are complete at the time of death. This will include clear identification of the patient.

7. Theatre staff must be aware of, and adhere to, the personal and cultural wishes of relatives as to jewellery or artefacts remaining on the patient. The nurse must identify and clearly record these articles.

8. It is essential that infection control and good hygiene are practised throughout all stages in this care, including transfer to the mortuary.

9. The senior nurse should ensure that the deceased patient is transferred to the mortuary as soon as possible following death. As a mark of respect, it is appropriate for a nurse to escort the deceased to the theatre suite exit.

10. The relatives should be given the opportunity to pay their last respects, if this is their preference. The provision of a private waiting area for relatives in the vicinity of the operating department is recommended. A quiet area should be made available to allow them to be alone with the deceased.

11. It is essential that operating department staff are given appropriate support following the death of a patient in the area.

Principles of Safe Practice in The Perioperative Environment

Patient Care- *Section 2*

PLANNING PATIENT CARE

Introduction

Planning care in the operating department involves care of the patient during the preoperative, intraoperative and postoperative stages. The assessment of patient needs is a continuous cycle which ensures that thorough, accurate and timely information for individualised patient care can be planned, implemented and evaluated. The importance of multi-professional care planning in the operating department is essential, not only for the well being of patients, but to contribute to the optimum and effective use of valuable resources. Where used, multi-professional care pathways will ensure that the patient receives the highest possible standard of care and the role of the nurse in theatre will be enhanced.

BIBLIOGRAPHY

Baldwin C 1993 Welcome visitor ... perioperative visit from a theatre nurse. Nursing Times. 89 (4) 44-46

Beddows J 1997 Alleviating preoperative anxiety in patients - a study. Nursing Standard. 11 (37) 35-38

Booth K 1992 PreOperative visiting : a step by step guide ...Part 1. British Journal of Theatre Nursing. 1 (7) 30-31.

Dodds F 1993 Access to the coping strategies : managing anxiety in elective surgical patients. Professional Nurse. 9 (1) 46-46, 48, 50

Droogan J Dickson R 1996 Preoperative patient instruction : is it effective? Nursing Standard. 10 (35) 32-33

Kane 1996 Sample perioperative care plan... standardised care plan. AORN Journal. 64 (5) 685

Martin D 1996 Preoperative visits to reduce patient anxiety : a study. Nursing Standard. 10 (23) 33-38

Ong B 1997 Patients approve of preoperative assessments. Nursing Times. (40) 57-59

Panda N 1996 Preoperative anxiety : effect of early or late position on the operating list. Anaesthesia. 51 (4) 344-346

Shirley M A 1993 Perioperative documentation : a generic OR care plan. AORN Journal. 57(6) 1431, 1434-1440

Webb R A 1995 Perioperative visiting from the perspective of the theatre nurse. British Journal of Nursing. 4 (19) 919-920, 922, 924-925 14-27

Wicker P 1995 Preoperative visiting - making it work. British Journal of Theatre Nursing. 5 (7) 16-19

White J John B 1997 The design and introduction of videos and leaflets. British Journal of Theatre Nursing. 7 (9) 9-13

Recommendations for Inclusion in Local Policy

Patient Assessment and Preoperative Visiting

It is imperative that the nurse appreciates that consent to surgery and subsequent information relating to consent are the responsibility of the consultant surgeon or his designated deputy. Any concern that a nurse has regarding a patient's understanding of a surgical procedure must be referred to the responsible clinician.

The preoperative visit and interview is a complex process which requires that the nurse has a high degree of communication and interpersonal skills as well as a sound clinical knowledge. Through the development of interviewing skills, the nurse can obtain relevant information from patients in order to plan care more individually and effectively.

The four main areas for effective patient assessment are:

1. Skills of the interviewer
2. The interview technique
3. The structure of the interview
4. The topics to be covered during the interview

1. The Skills of the Interviewer

a. Whilst observing and interviewing a patient the nurse must be aware of his or her own verbal and non verbal communication clues.

b. Good eye contact is necessary to build up trust - but do not stare as this is intimidating.

c. Smile and nod occasionally to encourage responses and to affirm what the patient is saying.

d. Face the patient and lean forward slightly to encourage openness, interest and trust.

e. Avoid halting speech, speech errors, using "uh", "OK" and other paralinguistic idiosyncrasies.

f. Ask only one question at a time and wait for the answer.

g. Avoid sending mixed messages. When verbal and non-verbal messages contradict each other the patient will usually believe the non-verbal.

h. Use normal every day English expressions rather than technical terms and adapt your dialect or accent to suit the patient if appropriate.

2. The Interview Technique

a. Prepare a checklist of questions pertinent to the care of the patient.

b. Obtain the patient's consent to be interviewed.

c. Ask only one question at a time.

d. Avoid "why" questions as this may imply that there is something wrong with the patient's behaviour in terms of the nurse's values

e. Be tactful and avoid emotionally charged words.

f. Refrain from over-emphasising a topic as the patient may become anxious.

g. Refrain from forcing answers.

h. Clarify what the patient is saying by using phrases such as 'do you mean....' or 'are you saying that ...'

i. Use the patient's own words to cue them in.

j. Use self-disclosure where appropriate as this encourages sharing.

3. The Structure of the Interview

a. Introduce yourself to the patient by name and title.

b. Patients will respond better when they know what is expected of them. Therefore inform the patient why the interview is being carried out and in what ways this interview is different from others and how it will help his or her care.

c. Select a time for the preoperative interview that is suitable to both parties.

d. Ensure privacy for the interview and minimal disturbance during the interview.

e. Ensure that the patient feels emotionally and physically comfortable.

f. Conclude the interview so that the patient feels involved in his or her care planning.

4. Topics to be covered during the interview

The following range of topics may be covered during the patient interview. A high proportion of the information will be available on the patient's ward care-plan and may be taken from there, or alternatively the one care-plan with a section for theatre assessment included may be used.

Suggested Topics:
Patient's perception of health
Nutritional and/or metabolic state
Activity and/or exercise abilities
Cognitive and emotional state
Role relationships
General appearance
Skin Condition
Physical findings
Cardiovascular problems
Respiratory problems
Gastro-intestinal problems
Neurological problems
Diagnostic investigations
Patient's knowledge deficit
Post-surgery expectations

Perioperative Care Planning Strategy

The following patient problems are identified to help in the construction of care plans and the setting of standards in the operating department can be divided into the following three phases.

1. Preoperative
2. Intraoperative
3. Postoperative

1. Preoperative Phase

Patient problems which are common to the preoperative phase are:

Fear related to potential outcome of surgery.
Anticipatory grieving due to loss of part of the body.

Alteration in nutrition.
Potential fluid volume deficit.
Sleep pattern disturbance.
Anticipatory anxiety due to unfamiliar environment and impending surgery.

2. Intraoperative Phase

Patient problems which are common to the intraoperative phase are:-

Potential alteration in respiratory function due to anaesthesia.
Potential fluid volume deficit due to blood loss during surgery.
Potential for injury due to decreased level of

consciousness.
Potential decrease in cardiac output due to anaesthesia, decreased mobility and venous pooling.
Potential for infection.

3. Postoperative Phase

Patient problems which are common to the postoperative phase are:-

Pain related to surgical procedure.
Potential injury due to returning level of consciousness.
Sensory-perceptual alterations due to returning level of consciousness.
Ineffective airway clearance due to retained secretions.

Preoperative Care - An example

Problem

Anticipatory anxiety due to unfamiliar surroundings and impending surgery.

Expected outcomes

The patient will be able to manage his or her anxiety by discussing a basic understanding of the surgical procedure and his or her own feelings about the surgery.

The patient will be able to discuss the reasons for nursing and medical interventions prior to surgery, the preoperative medication, the skin preparation, the journey to theatre and the waiting areas.

The patient will be kept warm and comfortable and environmental stimuli will be kept to a minimum.

Nursing Actions

Assess the patient's degree of anxiety, denial, depression or acceptance through preoperative interviewing. Encourage the patient to discuss concerns and questions about the procedures involved. Communicate unresolved questions or concern to the surgeon or anaesthetist.

Explain nursing procedures before implementing them.

Identify the patient when she/he comes to the operating department by name and reassure him/her that someone will be present at all times to care for him/her.

Position the patient with pillows and blankets as appropriate.

Organise activity so the anaesthetic room or theatre will be quiet before the patient is brought in and ensure that a trained theatre person is with him or her at all times.

Keep bright lights away from the patient's eyes and reduce the amount of threatening equipment as appropriate.

Intraoperative Care - An Example:

Problem

Potential for injury due to decreased level of consciousness.

Expected Outcomes

The patient will be free of injury to the skin from diathermy.

The patient will be free of injury from a foreign body being left in the wound.

The patient's temperature will be maintained within normal limit.

The patient will not experience a skin break, muscular-skeletal or nerve damage and skin will be free from redness or bruising.

Nursing Actions

Ensure that all safety checks are carried out on diathermy equipment prior to use.

Carry out a swab, needle and instrument count before, during and after the procedure.

Cover all parts of the patient's body not included in the operative site. Monitor body and room temperature throughout the procedure. Provide blood or fluid warmer. Where indicated, warm all fluids that will enter the body cavity. Place warm blankets on the patient after surgery.

Use appropriate lifting aids to prevent skin shearing. Align body in anatomically appropriate position. Pad bony prominences. Secure the patient as appropriate. Check for signs of pressure and friction at the end of the procedure.

Postoperative Care - An example:

Problem

Ineffective clearance of the airway due to retained secretions from anaesthesia.

Expected Outcomes

The patient will have normal and adequate respiratory function as demonstrated by:

> Rate of respiration.
> Depth of respiration.
> Rhythm of respiration.
> Clear breathing sounds which aerate all lung fields.

Nursing Actions

Assess respiratory rate, depth and pattern. Auscultate lungs for breathing sounds and observe for reactions.

Position patient on side, suctioning mouth and throat as appropriate. Carry out oral hygiene. Instruct patient on coughing and deep breathing as appropriate. Support wound site whilst coughing and allow rest periods.

Principles of Safe Practice in
The Perioperative Environment

Patient Care- *Section 2*

PREOPERATIVE PATIENT CARE

Introduction

This principle should be read in conjunction with the previous section, Planning Patient Care.

Preoperative care can be identified as the starting point for the planning of individual patient care before surgery. Research shows that patients who have been well informed before surgery have a better postoperative recovery and require less analgesia. Effective communication is essential. Pre-admission programmes and information packs have been proved to be useful, but whatever is used, effective communication is essential. Some hospitals arrange for adults and children to visit the perioperative environment before they are formally admitted for surgery. Close liaison is essential between theatre staff, ward staff and clinical staff to identify the patient's needs and plan care.

Preoperative information should include explanation of procedures, relating to transfer to, and arrival at, the operating department for surgery. It is recommended that the patient should not be left unattended during this phase.

BIBLIOGRAPHY

Allink K 1991 Preoperative Handover Surgical Nurse. 42 (2) 4, 5, 8-9

Beddows J 1997 Alleviating preoperative anxiety in patients : a study. Nursing Standard. 11 (37) 35-8

Booth K 1991 Preoperative Visiting. British Journal of Theatre Nursing. 1 (8) 6-7

Carter L Evans T 1996 Surgical Nurse. Preoperative visiting - a role for theatre nurses. British Journal of Nursing. 5 (4) 204, 206-7

Dodds F 1993 Access to the coping strategies : managing anxiety in elective surgical patients. Professional Nurse. 9 (1) 45-6, 48, 50

Flanagan M Fletcher J Hollingsworth H 1994. Preoperative shaving. Journal of Wound Care. 3 (7) 338

Hallstrom R Beck S L 1993 Implementation of the AORN Skin Shaving Standard. AORN Journal. 58 (3) 498-506

Jepsen O Bruttomesso K A 1993 The effectiveness of Preoperative Skin Preparations. AORN Journal. 58 (3) 477-483

Llewellyn-Thomas A 1990 Preoperative skin preparation. Surgical Nurse. 3 (2) 24-26

Martin D 1996 Preoperative visits to reduce patient anxiety: a study. Nursing Standard. 10 (23) 33-38

NATN 1998 Safeguards for Invasive Procedures. The Management of Risks. Harrogate, NATN

NATN 1998 Ethical Issues. Principles Of Safe Practice In The Perioperative Environment. Harrogate, NATN

NATN 1998 Departmental Organisation. Principles Of Safe Practice In The Perioperative Environment. Harrogate, NATN

NATN 1998 Surgical Preparation of the Patient. Principles Of Safe Practice In The Perioperative Environment. Harrogate, NATN

Recommendations for Inclusion in Local Policy

General Considerations

1. Accurate information about the patient in the preoperative stage will ensure that the theatre team is able to plan, and subsequently deliver, individual patient care.

2. Consideration and care should be given to patients who have communication difficulties, ie: sensory loss, language barriers or learning difficulties. The appropriate aids and/or interpreters should be made available to the patient as required.

3. Information on identification bands should be accurate and legible. The bands should be secured on the wrists and/or ankle in order that the patient may be identified at all times.

4. To give consent, the patient should be well informed about the operative procedure. **This is the primary responsibility of the medical staff**. If there is obvious confusion or misunderstanding, a member of the medical team should be asked to explain any discrepancy to the patient.

5. The consent form should be completed correctly, in accordance with the national guidelines. The operation site(s) should be clearly marked by the surgeon and should correspond with the information on the consent form and the operation list.

6. A clear record should be available of any medication administered to the patient. This should include the time of administration and dosage of all drugs given. Prescription cards must accompany the patient during his or her stay in the operating department in order that they are available for reference at all times.

7. It is essential that all relevant documentation, notes, laboratory results, X-rays, allergies and consent forms are available for use in the operating department.

8. Care should be taken in preparing the patient for surgery in order to promote wound healing and minimise the risk of infection.

    a. The bed or trolley used to transport the patient must be clean.

    b. Fresh bed linen and a clean operating gown are essential.

    c. The patient's skin should be clean. Consideration should be given to the use of bactericidal soap solution to clean the skin. Specific preventative measures may be required to prepare the operative site, eg: antiseptic spray to the knee area.

    d. Local policies and procedures related to the preoperative hair removal should be determined after consultation with infection control staff.

9. It is recommended that there is a close liaison with the ward staff to ensure that patients undergoing general anaesthesia are prevented from developing dehydration, due to excessive periods of preoperative fasting. Special considerations may be required to be taken into account, for example, intravenous fluid therapy for diabetic patients.

10. It is recommended that parents be allowed to escort their child to the operating department. They may support their child in the anaesthetic room at the discretion of the anaesthetist.

11. It is essential that sufficient members of staff are available to ensure the safety of the patient, and staff, during transfer.

    a. Trolleys and beds must have;

        i. The facility for head-down tilt.

        ii. Effective brakes.

        iii. Padded protection on bed or trolley sides to prevent injury to the patient.

b. Care must be taken to ensure that the patient is fully supported during transfer procedures in order to prevent injury. Consideration must be given to the use of transfer aids or mechanical hoists.

12. Qualified theatre staff must receive patients into the department and ensure that the accompanying documentation is in order and complete.

13. It is recommended that theatre personnel be aware of the legal implications of informed consent.

14. All patients must be under constant supervision following their arrival in the operating department.

Principles of Safe Practice in The Perioperative Environment

Patient Care- Section 2

POSTOPERATIVE CARE

Introduction

This section of the principles document will address the demanding role of caring for the patient in the postoperative environment. As with nursing in all areas of care, there is a need for recovery staff to stay updated in new surgical and anaesthetic procedures and technology, recognising the influence these may have on the patient in the immediate postoperative period. Postoperative visits allow nurses to evaluate their care and enable the quality of patient care to be maintained and developed at this stage.

BIBLIOGRAPHY

AAGBI 1993 The High Dependency Unit - Acute care in the Future. London, The Association of Anaesthetists of Great Britain and Ireland

AAGBI 1993 Immediate Postanaesthetic Recovery. London, The Association of Anaesthetists of Great Britain and Ireland

AAGBI 1994 Recommendations for Standards of Monitoring during Anaesthesia and Recovery. London, The Association of Anaesthetists of Great Britain and Ireland

Allin K 1991 Postoperative Handover (Handing over patients from the theatre nurse to the ward nurse). Surgical Nurse. 4 (3) 23-27

Brigden R J 1990 Operating Department Technique. Churchill Livingstone, London

Eltringham R Durkin M Andrews S Casey W 1998 Post-Anaesthetic Recovery - a practical approach. Springer-Verlag, London

Hunter D 1991 Relief through Teamwork (Establishing an acute pain team for postoperative patients). Nursing Times. April 35-36, 38

NATN 1998 Preoperative Patient Care. Principles Of Safe Practice In The Perioperative Environment. Harrogate, NATN

NATN 1998 Visitors to the Perioperative Environment. Principles Of Safe Practice In The Perioperative Environment. Harrogate, NATN

NATN 1998 Potential hazards to Staff. Principles Of Safe Practice In The Perioperative Environment. Harrogate, NATN

NATN 1998 Care of the Child. Principles Of Safe Practice In The Perioperative Environment. Harrogate, NATN

NHS Estates 1991 Health Building Note 26 Operating Department, HMSO

Mackintosh C Bowles S 1997 Evaluation of a Nurse-led acute pain service. Can clinical nurse specialists make a difference? Journal of Advanced Nursing. 25 (1) 30-37

Shade P 1992 Patient-controlled analgesia - can client education improve outcome? Journal of Advanced Nursing. 17 (4) 408-413

Tate S Cook H 1996 Postoperative nausea and vomiting 1: physiology and aetiology. British Journal of Nursing. 5 (16) 962, 964, 966

Tate S Cook H 1996 Postoperative nausea and vomiting 2: management and treatment. British Journal of Nursing. 5 (17) 1032-1037

Recommendations for Inclusion in Local Policy

There are four areas for consideration:-

1. Design
2. Environment
3. Equipment
4. Nursing

1. Design

a. It is recommended that the recovery area is located near to the theatre reception area to allow free access of patients to and from wards.

b. The DOH (1989), recommends that a ratio of two bed spaces per operating room are allocated in the recovery area. It is important however, that consideration is given to the number of cases per session, the average recovery time of each patient and the arrangements for transporting patients for the area, when bed ratios are identified.

c. Bed space area should comply with the requirement for dealing with an emergency situation.

d. A central station should be position in order to allow observation of the whole recovery area.

e. Permanent screens must not be erected as these obstruct the total observation of patients.

f. Facilities for storage of clean and sterile equipment should be available and subject to local operational policies, eg; storage of drugs.

g. Access to utility rooms and sluice facilities are required.

h. i. It is essential that the recovery room is fully equipped to deal with emergency resuscitation, whilst ensuring immediate access to this equipment from all parts of the recovery area.

   ii. A system of summoning aid in the event of an emergency must be available. This must include the provision of alarm bells.

   iii. It is recommended that an individual anaesthetist is identified who is available at all times during a session, should an emergency occur.

j. The decor should be pleasant and comply with regulations to allow cleaning to take place in accordance with a planned preventative maintenance programme.

k. If the recovery area is used for patients who have undergone local and general anaesthetic procedures, consideration should be given to the placement of patients who are awake and fully orientated to their surroundings.

l. Recommendations to recover adult and paediatric patients in a separate environment should be taken into account.

2. Environment

a. The recovery area should be kept clean at all times.

b. The room temperatures should be maintained between 19-22 degrees celsius and should be free from draughts.

c. There should be a positive pressure ventilation facility in the recovery area to ensure that exhaled anaesthetic gases are removed effectively.

d. In order to promote a peaceful recovery for postoperative patients, noise levels should be controlled.

e. Lighting should allow for effective patient observation but should be conducive to patient comfort.

f. Recovery staff should be aware of safe practice related to storage of equipment, the handling of blood and bodily fluids and disposal of contaminated waste.

3. Equipment

a. Each bed space must be equipped with:-

   i. Oxygen and suction facilities.

   ii. Electric sockets.

   iii. Individual lamp.

   iv. Sphygmomanometer and stethoscope.

   v. monitoring equipment for the observation of:-

   > electrocardiograph
   > pulse oximetry
   > non-invasive blood pressure
   > arterial pressure
   > central venous pressure

b. The recovery bed or trolley, must have an operational two way tilt facility. Trolleys should have padded sides.

c. Emergency equipment must be accessible and should include that required for:-

   > endotracheal intubation
   > defibrillation
   > tracheotomy
   > malignant hyperpyrexia
   > anaphylaxis

d. Equipment should be available to deal with inadvertent hypothermia.

e. It is essential that all equipment in recovery is in working order and that it is checked daily. Any faulty equipment should be replaced and sent for repair immediately.

4. Nursing

1. Nurses working in the recovery area must possesses the knowledge and understanding of the implications of the surgery the patient has undergone and the complications which can be expected.

2. They must be competent in airway management.

3. They must be competent in assessing the patient's condition and in administering pain relief as necessary and in accordance with local policy.

4. They must be competent in caring for the ventilated patient in accordance with local policy.

5. If children are to be recovered in the area, then a paediatric nurse should be a member of the team or the area have access to advice of a qualified paediatric nurse (RSCN) in accordance with local policy.

Principles of Safe Practice in The Perioperative Environment

Patient Care- *Section 2*

CARE OF THE PATIENT UNDERGOING SURGERY IN THE DAY CARE SETTING

Introduction

Day surgery is defined as surgery performed on a patient who is admitted for investigation or operation on a planned non-resident basis, and who requires facilities for recovery in a ward or unit.

This definition excludes minor operative procedures undertaken on a walk-in basis, in out-patient or accident and emergency departments.

It is recommended that day surgery be provided in the environment of a fully equipped general hospital (Royal College of Surgeons 1992).

Day surgical care should not be regarded as a sub-speciality of surgery. It is an appropriate surgery performed on a day basis from within, preferably, a dedicated Day Surgery Unit. It therefore requires the same facilities as those available for in-patient surgery.

Day surgical nursing care should be of the same high standard as in-patient care. It is essential to provide adequate information to patients who will be required to arrive prepared for same-day surgery and who are expected to care for themselves with only minimal, non-expert assistance within hours of surgical intervention and the administration of general, local, regional anaesthesia or sedation.

Day surgical treatment should not be a cheap option. Surgery, anaesthesia and nursing care must only be carried out by senior personnel to ensure a swift, safe and sympathetic progress through an area dedicated solely to the care of day surgical patients, so that they will not need to be treated as secondary to patients who require more major or emergency treatment in an acute situation.

BIBLIOGRAPHY

AAGBI 1994 Day Case Surgery. Association of Anaesthetists of Great Britain and Ireland, London

AORN 1990 Perioperative Nursing Documentation. Denver, AORN Inc

AORN, 1991 Standards and Recommended Practices for Perioperative Nursing. Denver, AORN Inc.

Audit Commission 1990 "A Short Cut to Better Services", Day Surgery in England and Wales. HMSO, London

Bates J 1994 Reducing fast times in paediatric day surgery. Nursing Times. 90 (48) 38-39

Beaumont S 1997 Preoperative Assessment for Day Case Surgery: A Patient Centred Service. British Journal of Theatre Nurses. 7 (9) 9, 12-13

Brown A Duxby J 1997 Day Surgery - Communication and Interviewing Skills. British Journal of Theatre Nursing. 7 (3) 10, 12, 14-15

DOH 1991 Day Surgery Making it Happen. Value for Money Unit, London, HMSO

Green D 1995 Patient assessment for day surgery. British Journal of Theatre Nursing. 5 (1) 10-12

Knowles J 1997 Preassessment of the Day Surgery Patient. British Journal of Theatre Nursing. 7 (3) 16-18

NATN 1998 Surgical Preparation of the Patient for Surgery. Principles Of Safe Practice In The Perioperative Environment. Harrogate, NATN

Neasham J 1996 Nurse Led Pre-Assessment Clinic. British Journal of Theatre Nursing. 6 (8) 5, 8-10

Mitchell M 1997 Patients' perceptions of preoperative preparation for day surgery. Advanced Journal of Nursing. 26 (2) 356-363

Reid J H 1997 Meeting the informational needs of patients in a day surgery setting - An exploratory study. British Journal of Theatre Nursing. 7 (3) 19-24

West B J M Lyons M H 1995 Day Surgery: Cheap option or challenge to care? British Journal of Theatre Nursing. 5 (1) 5-8

Young S Munro F 1995 Some patient preoperative anxieties in day surgery. Journal - One Day Surgery. Autumn 5 (2) 21-22

Recommendations for Inclusion in Local Policy

1. Patient selection
2. Pre admission assessment and preparation
3. Admission
4. Perioperative care
5. Evaluation and audit

1. Patient Selection

Quality care and safe nursing practice can only be effective when patients are rigorously and suitably selected for day surgical care. Suitable selection is the responsibility of the referring general practitioner and consultant surgeon at out patient consultation. Advice should also be sought from consultant anaesthetists practising in day surgery. The following are basic guide lines.

a. All patients must be escorted home accompanied by a responsible and informed adult.

b. All patients must be adequately supervised during their recovery at home for a minimum period of 24 hours. The 24 hour period of restriction will need to be extended to 48 hours when benzodiazepines, sedatives or opioids have been administered in conjunction with general, regional or local anaesthesia.

c. Patients must have suitable home conditions with adequate toilet facilities.

d. Anxious or phobic patients may benefit from a night in hospital if pre-medication is considered desirable.

e. Over-anxious parents may prefer professional support in hospital to assist in the care of their child in the immediate postoperative period.

f. Physiological fitness should be considered, rather than a strictly applied chronological age-limit. It is necessary to screen all patients for physiological suitability regardless of age.

g. No operative procedure should be performed if it carries a risk of excessive postoperative pain, haemorrhage or prolonged immobility. Community assistance may be sought for follow up arrangements and wound dressing. It is the responsibility of the day surgery nurse to liaise with community services to arrange follow up care.

h. Patients with cardiovascular, respiratory diseases, diabetes and gross obesity are not suitable to be treated as day cases. Borderline cases may be referred to the relevant anaesthetist.

i. The patient should have access to a telephone for advice and for an emergency.

j. Distances to be travelled postoperatively should not exceed one hour.

2. Pre-Admission Assessment and Preparation

a. All patients receiving appointments for day surgical treatment must be reassessed by suitably experienced nursing staff before admission to ensure that borderline cases are referred to the relevant anaesthetist.

b. Detailed verbal information about operative procedure, mode of anaesthetic, possible postoperative restrictions and symptoms, must be explained before admission date. The day surgery nurse should be assured that informed consent for operation has been obtained by clinicians.

c. All patients should receive written preoperative instructions with regard to social arrangements, preparation for surgery (ie: fasting) and the nature of their anaesthetic and surgical treatment. Written information about attendance time, anticipated waiting time and expected sequence of events, discharge time and car parking arrangements should be provided at initial assessment interview.

d. Assessment and future plan of care be initiated. Documentation of health status prior to the day of surgery, preferably following outpatient visit, will ensure that preoperative investigations (ie: Hb, X-ray) may be completed before admission date.

3. Admission

a. Initial establishment of patient/nurse rapport is essential immediately on admission. Any undue anxiety or adverse psychological state detrimental to favourable outcome will need to be resolved prior to administration of the chosen anaesthetic and before surgical intervention. Pre-medication is not normally indicated for day surgical procedures, thus nursing care will involve the strategic use of highly refined communication skills, sensory information and verbal and non-verbal support to reduce anxiety.

b. Any alteration in current health status, social arrangements or discharge plan must be documented and communicated to the relevant clinicians prior to treatment. All day surgery patients undergo the same careful preparations for surgery as do their in patient counterparts (see this section on the Surgical Preparation of the Patient for Surgery).

c. Allergic reactions, base-line monitoring, physiological abnormalities, patient identity, suitable skin preparation and electrosurgery precautions are carefully documented and communicated to the perioperative environment personnel.

4. Perioperative Care

a. The day surgery nurse must possess a sound knowledge of all forms of anaesthesia, their adverse reactions and potential physiological effects and the potential minor sequelae which patients may experience regardless of the type of anaesthetic administered. All patients are monitored for reaction to anaesthetic drugs throughout and immediately after completion of procedure. Basic observations should include blood pressure, heart rate and rhythm, respiratory rate, oxygen saturation, skin condition and mental state.

b. The same rigorous adherence applies to standard and safe nursing practice in the day surgery operating theatre as is recommended for all operating theatres. Infection control, manipulation of the environment, surgical preparation of the patient, safe positioning, skin preparation aseptic technique, swab, instrument and needle counts must be of uniform standard and carried out in accordance with local policy.

c. Privacy, dignity and confidentiality of all day surgery patients must be preserved at all times. No information must be disclosed to relatives escorts or friends without prior permission from the patient. Examination of patients while under the effect of general anaesthesia by medical students must be regulated and prior written consent obtained from the patient.

d. Day care surgery may potentially be conducted under general, regional or local anaesthetic. Nurses caring for these patients in the recovery phase should be competent in the following skills:-

   i. Total support of the unconscious patient.

   ii. Management of the airway and extubation.

   iii. Monitoring levels of consciousness and minimising disorientation.

   iv. Assessing and treating post operative pain.

   v. Treating nausea and vomiting.

   vi. Managing the respiratory or cardiac emergency.

   vii. Performing cardio-pulmonary resuscitation.

e. Discharge criteria should be set in consultation with medical practitioners. If the day surgery nurse discharges the patient it will be necessary to ensure that patients are adequately informed, in writing and verbally, as to the nature of the operative procedure, anticipated postoperative progress and future follow-up arrangements and that:-

   i. Vital signs have returned to base line parameters.

   ii. Fluids can be tolerated and patient has voided.

   iii. Pain is controlled and analgesics supplied.

   iv. Haemorrhage or wound haematoma is absent.

   v. Mobility aids are provided as necessary.

   vi. Follow up and community care arrangements are made.

   vii. Responsible and informed escort is available.

   viii. Social support and close supervision is available for 24 hours following general anaesthesia.

   ix. Guidelines should be incorporated into local policy for patients who may be require to be admitted for in-patient care.

5. Evaluation and Audit

a. Continuous monitoring and evaluation of the quality of surgical treatment, anaesthetic agent, nursing care and postoperative self-management and pain control can be assessed by the use of questionnaires, postoperative phone calls, re-admission rates and incidence of infection or complications at follow up consultation and by canvassing community personnel. Patient and carer satisfaction can be ascertained in a similar fashion.

b. Review of the adequacy of written and verbal information and consultation with other health professionals will be an ongoing commitment in order to adapt and improve upon the information offered and to ensure full understanding of day surgical patients knowledge.

c. Collection of relevant statistics, budgetary control and costings are important aspects of day surgical audit.

Principles of Safe Practice in The Perioperative Environment

Patient Care- *Section 2*

INADVERTENT HYPOTHERMIA RELATED TO THE SURGICAL PATIENT

Introduction

The healthy body maintains its own natural temperature. This is achieved by the hypothalamus in conjunction with the sympathetic nervous system. Changes in body temperature can be identified by the following:-

- an increase or decrease in metabolic rate
- shivering
- vasoconstriction or vasodilatation which alters the blood supply to the skin

Definition of Hypothermia

Hypothermia is a decrease of the body's core temperature to below the normal limits of 36 - 38 C

There are three stages of hypothermia:-

Mild:	33 - 35.5 C
Moderate:	30-33 C
Severe:	Below 30 C

Inadvertent Hypothermia

This is the accidental lowering of a patient's body temperature - in this case during surgery.

There are two groups of contributing factors to inadvertent hypothermia.

1. Intrinsic factors: - those that are related to the surgical or anaesthetic process:

Lack of food - preoperative fasting for longer than necessary
Immobility
Preoperative drugs
Nervousness, anxiety
Anaesthetics, including regional blocks
Loss of shivering process
Type of surgery - extensive exposure of wound
Age of patient
Physical condition of patient

2. Extrinsic Factors - those which can be identified and remedied

Lack of clothing (for example, a patient wearing a gown only)
Lack of adequate bedding (for example, a patient covered with blanket only)
Draughty areas (corridors, lifts, reception areas, etc)
Cold environment in theatre
Thinness of surgical drapes used alone
Non-humidified fluids (for example, blood)
Cold irrigation fluids (for example, during transurethral resection of prostate)
Unnecessary exposure of patients
Non-use of warming equipment

A combination of these factors can lead to inadvertent hypothermia on the day of surgery.

There is evidence that some patients are more susceptible to inadvertent hypothermia than others. Risk factors should be assessed on an individual patient basis.

Those patients most at risk are:-

i. The very young.

ii. The very elderly.

iii. Cachetic or emaciated patients.

iv. Patients with pre-existing endocrine disorders.

v. Paralysed and anaesthetised patients.

The implications for a patient developing inadvertent hypothermia can be profound and can markedly affect their metabolism of anaesthetic drugs, leading to possible subsequent periods of apnoea in the postoperative period.

BIBLIOGRAPHY

Andrews A J 1990 Inadvertent Hypothermia. AORN Journal. 52 (5) 987-991

Blackburn E 1994 Prevention of Hypothermia during Anaesthesia. British Journal of Theatre Nursing. 4 (8) 9-13

Brook-Brunn J A 1994 Commentary on Prevention of Intraoperative hypothermia by preoperative skin surface warming. AACN Nursing Scan in Critical Care. 4 (1) 29 Jan-Dec

Closs J 1992 Monitoring the body temperature of surgical patients. Surgical Nurse. 5 (1) 12-16

Dennison D 1995 Thermal regulation of patients during the preoperative period. AORN Journal. 61 (5) 827-828

DOH 1991 Hazard Warning - Misuse of Laboratory Water Bath for Warming Blood for Transfusions. HC(91)18

DOH 1991 Safety Action Bulletin - Misuse of Commercially Available Microwave Appliances (Fluids for Clinical Administration), SAB(91)45

Ellis-Stoll C C Anderson C Cantu L G Englert S J Carlile W E 1996 Effect of continuously warmed IV fluids on intraoperative hypothermia. AORN Journal. 63 (3) 599-600, 602-606

Fox J 1993 Chilling Facts. Nursing Times. 89 (41) 76-80

Imrie M Hall G 1990 Body Temperature and Anaesthesia. British Journal of Anaesthetics. 64, 346-354

McNeil B A 1998 Addressing the Problems of Inadvertent Hypothermia in Surgical Patients Part 1 - Addressing the Issues. British Journal of Theatre Nursing. 8 (4) 8-14

McNeil B A 1998 Addressing the Problems of Inadvertent Hypothermia in Surgical Patients Part 2 - Self learning package. British Journal of Theatre Nursing. 8 (4) 8-14

Moddeman G 1991 The Elderly Surgical Patient - a high risk of hypothermia. AORN Journal. 53 (5) 1270-1272

Ouellette R G 1994 Perioperative Hypothermia. Current Reviews for Nurse Anaesthetists. 16 (22) 195-200

Pudner M 1992 Inadvertent Hypothermia. Technic. Issue 106, 10-11

Surkitt-Parr M 1992 Hypothermia in Surgical Patients. British Journal of Nursing. 1 (11) 539-545

Touzeau P F 1994 The Big Chill - inadvertent hypothermia. ACORN Journal. 7 (4) 26-28

Tudor M 1994 Scaling of the patients temperature. Part 2. British Journal of Theatre Nursing. 3 (12) 14-15

Anonymous 1997 Keeping patients normothermic during an operation. Seminars in Perioperative Nursing. 6 (1) 44-8

Recommendations for Inclusion in Local Policy

The two areas for consideration are:

1.   Preoperative measures
2.   Intraoperative measures

1. Preoperative Measures

a.   Patients should be fasted for no longer than local preoperative fasting regimes stipulate.

b.   Care must be taken to ensure that patients are comfortable with their temperature at all times and where necessary, adequate bed covering should be provided.

c.   The ritual of making theatre bedding packs should be examined carefully. The emphasis of the local procedure must be to ensure patient comfort at all times.

2. Intraoperative Measures

a.   i.   The environmental temperature in the theatre should be closely monitored and subsidiary equipment used to enhance it if required.

ii.   Theatre doors should be kept closed **at all times.** Access to theatre should be restricted in order to maintain room temperature and reduce draughts.

iii.   Particular care should be taken when caring for infants and neonates who lose heat rapidly. In such cases the theatre temperature should be raised to 27.5C in order to maintain the infant's body temperature.

iv.   When overhead radiant heating is in use, it should be positioned more than 24" above the patient.

b.   It is essential that the patient is kept covered **at all times.**

The patient should be exposed for a minimum time only:-

during positioning
prior to 'prepping'
following surgery

c.   All fluids to be used during anaesthetic or surgical procedures should be warmed before use. These include:-

intravenous fluids,
irrigation fluids and washout fluids,
saline for abdominal packs.

d.   All anaesthetic gases should be humidified.

e.   Heated mattresses and blankets should be used as necessary on the operating table and on patients' beds/cots in readiness for transfer following surgery. Convector heaters may be used where feasible. Thermal blankets, leggings etc. can be used where they don't interfere with the surgical field.

f.   Incubators should be left on to maintain optimum temperature.

g.   Where body heat has been lost during surgery, it is essential that where expediency allows, the patients' temperature is allowed to return to the appropriate range before he or she leaves theatre.

h.   It is important to monitor and record the temperature of all patients undergoing major surgery, the elderly patient and other patients at risk for inadvertent hypothermia.

In reception area of anaesthetic room.
In theatre.
In recovery.

Action should be taken as necessary.

Principles of Safe Practice in The Perioperative Environment

Patient Care- *Section 2*

CARE OF PATIENTS UNDERGOING ANAESTHETIC PROCEDURES

Introduction

Safe patient care in the anaesthetic area starts ideally with preoperative care in the surgical ward setting. It is well documented that patient's anxiety levels are reduced when they are well informed and have met staff involved in their care. The assessment, planning, evaluation and documentation of care is essential for the patient's well-being, however the opportunity for anaesthetic staff to assess the patient preoperatively is not always possible or attainable given the working demands of the operating department. In such circumstances where a preoperative assessment has not been carried out, the importance of good communication skills and an awareness of patient's needs are vital.

Maintaining a safe environment and current clinical practice with regard to the checking of equipment within a framework of infection control guidelines, ensures a holistic approach to safe practice.

The patient undergoing an anaesthetic intervention requires individual support at all times. Many operative departments recognise the need for a nominated nurse to provide this support for patients in the anaesthetic room. **When preparing local policies, it should be remembered that this principle relates to all others within the document and should not be considered in isolation.**

Within this principle, staff who are recognised as holding relevant anaesthetic support qualification will be referred to as "qualified anaesthetic staff".

BIBLIOGRAPHY

AAGBI 1988 Assistance for the Anaesthetist. London, Association of Anaesthetists of Great Britain and Ireland

AAGBI 1989 Efficiency of Theatre Services. London, Association of Anaesthetists of Great Britain and Ireland

AAGBI 1990 Checklists for Anaesthetic Machines. London, Association of Anaesthetists of Great Britain and Ireland

AAGBI 1991 The role of the Anaesthetist in the Emergency Services. London, Association of Anaesthetists of Great Britain and Ireland

AAGBI 1992 Immediate Post-Anaesthetic Recovery. London, Association of Anaesthetists of Great Britain and Ireland

AAGBI 1994 Recommendations for Standards of Monitoring during Anaesthesia and Recovery. London, Association of Anaesthetists of Great Britain and Ireland

Carter L Evans T 1996 Surgical Nurse. Preoperative visiting : a role for theatre nurses. British Journal of Nursing. 5 (4) 919-920, 922, 924-925.

Dodds F 1993 Access to the coping strategies : Managing anxiety in elective patients. Professional Nurse. 9 (1) 45-46, 48, 50

Morrison P Burnard P 1991 Caring and Communications. Basingstoke, Macmillan Education Ltd.

NATN 1998 Education and Training. Principles Of Safe Practice In The Perioperative Environment. Harrogate, NATN

NATN 1998 Fire. Principles Of Safe Practice In The Perioperative Environment. Harrogate, NATN

NATN 1998 Infection Control. Principles Of Safe Practice In The Perioperative Environment. Harrogate, NATN

NATN 1998 Potential Hazards to Staff. Principles Of Safe Practice In The Perioperative Environment. Harrogate, NATN

NATN 1998 Management. Principles Of Safe Practice In The Perioperative Environment. Harrogate, NATN

NATN 1998 Planning Patient Care. Principles Of Safe Practice In The Perioperative Environment. Harrogate, NATN

NATN 1998 Pre-Operative Patient Care. Principles Of Safe Practice In The Perioperative Environment. Harrogate, NATN

NATN 1998. The Safeguards for Invasive Procedures : The Management of Risks. Harrogate, NATN

NATN 1998 Visitors to the Perioperative Environment. Principles Of Safe Practice In The Perioperative Environment. Harrogate, NATN

NATN 1998 Aseptic Technique. Principles Of Safe Practice In The Perioperative Environment. Harrogate, NATN

NATN 1998 Procedures Related to Organ Donation. Principles Of Safe Practice In The Perioperative Environment. Harrogate, NATN

Webb R A 1995 Preoperative visiting from the perspective of the theatre nurse. British Journal of Nursing. 4 (16) 919-920, 922, 924-925

Recommendations for Inclusion in Local Policy

The five main areas for consideration when preparing local policies are:-

1. Personnel Issues
2. Patient Care
3. Preparation and Maintenance of Anaesthetic Equipment
4. Infection Control/Clinical Practice
5. Patient Safeguards

1. Personnel Issues

a. It is essential that all staff who work in the anaesthetic room and undertake direct patient care hold a professional qualification recognised in that care setting and related to this area of care.

b. It is essential that qualified anaesthetic staff take every opportunity to keep up-to-date with current and relevant professional knowledge and are able to evaluate its use in patient care.

c. All qualified anaesthetic staff must accept responsibility for their own continuing personal and professional development.

2. Patient Care

a. Qualified anaesthetic staff must be aware of the psychological, social and cultural factors which influence the patient's response to illness and disease. It is essential that staff are able to develop supportive and understanding relationships with patients awaiting anaesthetic intervention by demonstrating understanding of particular needs.

b. It is essential that all qualified anaesthetic staff should understand the importance of good inter-personal and communication skills with particular reference to:-

i. The use/non use of face masks.

ii. The effects of hearing or visual loss.

iii. The importance of effective and instrumental touch.

iv. Facial expression and the importance of non-verbal clues.

v. The giving of information to patients.

c. It is essential that all qualified anaesthetic staff must be able to demonstrate skills in assessment, planning, implementation and evaluation of patient care and document this information accordingly.

3. Preparation and Maintenance of Anaesthetic Equipment

a. It is essential that all routine safety checks on anaesthetic equipment are carried out in accordance with the guidelines issued by the Association of Anaesthetists of Great Britain and Ireland.

b. All anaesthetic equipment must be checked, prepared and demonstrated as functional before induction of anaesthesia is commenced.

c. All anaesthetic equipment must undergo regular maintenance checks by medical engineers and/or service contractors in accordance with national guidelines and local policies and maintenance should be registered accordingly.

d. Qualified anaesthetic staff must be aware of the relative costs of anaesthetic equipment and the need for reasonable economy in its preparation, use and maintenance.

4. Infection Control/Clinical Practice

a. In order to ensure control of infection, it is essential to maintain a high standard of asepsis in the anaesthetic room at all times. All staff must be encouraged to apply and maintain this standard rigorously.

b. Clear guidelines must be in place for the effective disinfection and sterilisation of anaesthetic equipment and these must be strictly observed at all times. It will be necessary to refer to the manufacturer's guidelines and the local infection control team when developing local policy.

c. Disposable receptacles for anaesthetic equipment are recommended for each individual patient. Where non-disposable receptacles are used, it is essential that these are autoclavable and processed accordingly for **each** patient.

d. Specific and detailed protocols should be available which relate to clinical anaesthetic procedures, for example, epidural technique.

5. Patient Safeguards

a. Qualified anaesthetic staff must be aware of potential hazards to patients and take all necessary precautions to prevent any untoward incidents related to environmental safety. National guidelines and local policies must be adhered to at all times, in particular with regard to:-

   i. Explosions and fire.

   ii. Electrical and radiation hazards.

   iii. Pollution.

   iv. Chemical substances.

b. It is essential that careful identification and checking procedures are carried out with regard to each individual patient, the accompanying documentation and sites of operation. The checks must be conducted:-

   i. when sending for the patient from the ward.

   ii. when the patient arrives in the operating department.

   iii. in the anaesthetic room prior to induction.

   iv. in the theatre prior to surgery.

c. Qualified anaesthetic staff must be competent in identifying and minimising potential hazards to unconscious and sedated patients.

d. Patients must be supported at all times by a nominated staff member when awaiting induction of anaesthesia.

e. It is essential that the standard procedures for the identification, storage, security and administration of drugs, intravenous fluids and blood products are rigorously applied at all times by qualified anaesthetic staff, in line with local policies and procedures.

f. All anaesthetic drugs must be drawn up by a qualified medical practitioner or by appropriately trained anaesthetic personnel where local policy permits.

i. Drugs should be placed in a disposable receptacle and remain with the patient throughout surgery prior to disposal at the end of the procedure.

ii. During a critical incident qualified anaesthetic staff may be required to administer drugs for intravenous use. This should be done only under the direct supervision of a qualified medical practitioner.

Principles of Safe Practice in The Perioperative Environment

Patient Care- *Section 2*

CARE OF THE CHILD

Introduction

Children and their parents or carers who receive advance preparation for hospital admission, often cope better with the events that surround operation day. Preparation of children prior to admission for surgery can help reduce unnecessary fear, distress and anxiety and creates a more positive and less traumatic hospital and theatre experience.

Pre-admission hospital visits, Saturday clubs, hospital information booklets, preparation videos in outpatient clinics, preoperative play and preoperative visiting on wards by perioperative staff, all assist in the psychological and educational preparation for surgery.

The parent or carer is a valued member of the child care team and should be encouraged to share in the child's hospital care. Providing overnight accommodation for them in hospital can help to make life easier for the parent or carer during a potentially stressful time.

Children have different emotional and physical needs and require appropriately trained staff who are able to assess and meet their needs.

The government has acknowledged the special needs of children and their families. The Children's Act (1989) along with the Clothier Report on the Allitt Inquiry have all been instrumental in ensuring that child care is constantly under review.

In addition, this principle should be read in conjunction with the principles entitled Postoperative Patient Care, Care of the Patient Undergoing Day Surgery, Inadvertent Hypothermia related to the Surgical Patient, Visitors to the Perioperative Environment and the NATN document 'Nursing the

Paediatric patient in the Adult Perioperative Environment'. This paediatric section will outline the preparation of children for surgery and suggest guidelines in the care of children in the operating department.

BIBLIOGRAPHY

Adams J 1992 Devising Booklets for Parents. Cascade. 1 (5), 7

Alderson P 1992 Choosing for Children Parent's Consent to Surgery. Milton Keynes, Oxford University Press

Alderson P 1992 Consent to Surgery (particularly in relation to children). Hospital Update. 18 (7) 529-532

Allitt Enquiry 1994 Clinical Supervision for Nursing and Health Visiting Professionals. London, DOH

Bailey R C 1992 Children in Theatre : Meeting Their Needs. British Journal of Theatre Nursing. 2 (3) 4-8.

Bourne A 1992 A Paediatric Day Service. British Journal of Theatre Nursing. 2 (3) 17

Brill J 1992 Control of Pain. Critical Care Clinics. 8 (1) 203-218

Charles-Edwards I Casey A 1992 Parental Involvement and Voluntary Consent Paediatric Nursing. 4 (1) 16-18

Children Act 1989

Dolan A 1993 A Day in the Life of a Hospital Play Specialist. British Journal of Theatre Nursing. 3 (3) 31-32

Donnelly J 1992 The Children's Act - A Brief Report. British Journal of Theatre Nursing. 2 (3) 12-13

Gillies M 1993 Postoperative Pain in the Child - literature review. Journal of Clinical Nursing. (1) 5-10

Glasper A Burge D 1992 Developing Family Information leaflets. Nursing Standard. 6 (25) 24-27

May L 1992 reducing Pain and Anxiety in Children. Nursing Standard. 6 (44) 25-28

Murray B 1992 Natalie: A Patient Case Study. British Journal of Theatre Nursing. 2 (3) 9-10

NATN 1996 Nursing the Paediatric Patient in the Adult Perioperative Environment. Harrogate, NATN

NATN 1998 Patient Care. Principles Of Safe Practice In The Perioperative Environment. Harrogate, NATN

NATN 1998 Visitors to the Perioperative Environment. Principles Of Safe Practice In The Perioperative Environment. Harrogate, NATN

Norris E 1992 Care of the Paediatric Day Surgery Patient. British Journal of Nursing. 1 (11) 547-551

Nursing Standard Supplement, 1993 Managing Children in Pain 10 1(25)

O'Neill S 1992 Children in Recovery. Nursing Times. 88 (41) 68-70

Peutrell J Wolf A 1992 Pain Relief in Children - Postoperative Pain Relief in Neonates and Children. British Journal of Hospital Medicine. 47 (4) 289-293

Rushton K Elliot B 1992 Transportation of Children on Trolleys. Paediatric Nursing. 4 (5) 24-27

White A Crawford J 1992 Paediatric Day Surgery. Nursing Times. 88 (39) 43-45

Children's Books about Hospital

Donnelly J 1992 Teddy Goes to Hospital. Countrywide Ltd.

Recommendations for Inclusion in Local Policy

The main areas for consideration are:-

1. The Preparation of children for surgery
2. Admission to the operating department
3. Non-threatening perioperative environment
4. Arrival in the anaesthetic room.
5. The child in theatre
6. Postoperative and recovery room care.

1. Preparation of the Child for Surgery

a. Children need the support on their parents or carers on operation day as this helps to reduce the unnecessary anxiety and distress. Parents or carers should be encouraged to share in all aspects of their children's hospital care.

b. Children should be encouraged to bring one or two of their favourite toys and books into hospital. Parents or carers should not worry if their child still needs their favourite blanket or soother or that these might look a bit worn or old. The child will feel more secure and often settle more easily. Children should also be allowed to bring their favourite toy or soother to theatre.

c. **Preoperative preparation is essential.** Parents or carers and the child should have an understanding of basic procedures of the operation day and be given the opportunity to ask questions. In addition to the visit by the surgeon and anaesthetist, a preoperative visit from a trained member of the perioperative staff who will be caring for that particular child in theatre is beneficial.

d. If it is not possible for the child to wear his own clothing to come to theatre, then patterned coloured pyjamas or gown should be available.

e. Children who have not had a pre-medication could be given a choice in how they wish to travel to theatre, for example, walking with their parent or carer, riding a toy or being carried, as an alternative to the theatre trolley.

f. The use of local anaesthetic cream has considerably reduced the fear associated with injections and needles and helps make the induction of anaesthesia a smoother and more comfortable procedure for the child.

2. Admission to the Operating Department

a. A parent or familiar adult should be welcome to accompanying the child into the anaesthetic room if they so wish. This helps to maintain the reassurance and smoothness of the child's operation day and is less traumatic for the child. At this point the child should never feel that they have been handed over to strangers or suddenly feel abandoned by their parent or carer, in who they have complete trust. It is important that the hospital has an agreed policy that parents or carers can escort their child into the anaesthetic room, providing the anaesthetist is in agreement and there are no clinical implications for the parent or carer not being present. Parents or carers should be made aware of this policy as early as possible and information about the policy can be included in the preoperative preparations thus avoiding unnecessary worry and distress.

3. Non-Threatening Perioperative Environment

a. Colourful walls, ceilings, pictures, posters, children's paintings, mobiles, toys, patterned cushioned trolley sides, patterned theatre gowns and pyjamas all help reduce anxiety and create a distraction for children and parents or carers in hospital and in the perioperative environment. In addition, these items create a relaxed atmosphere for adult patients.

b. Good staff attitudes are very important and parents or carers should be welcomed to theatre and children greeted to their level of maturity.

c. A parent or carer waiting area should be provided near the operating department.

d. Consideration should be given to the reception and recovery areas to ensure that children are not exposed to seriously ill or injured adults. Wherever possible, children should be nursed in a specifically designated area.

4. Arrival in the Anaesthetic Room

a. Both child and their parent or carer should be welcomed.

b. As with any patient, care is required to ensure that:-

   i. Only necessary equipment is left in the anaesthetic room.

   ii. Privacy and dignity is maintained at all times with no unnecessary removal of the child's clothing.

   iii. Staff numbers in the anaesthetic room should be kept to a minimum.

   iv. Doors should be kept shut at all times.

   v. There should be no sudden noises

c. A nurse or other specifically identified staff member should be available to escort the parent or carer out of the operating department, and where possible back to the ward, once the child is asleep.

5. The Child in Theatre

a. As with all parents, before the child arrives in theatre, a suitable environment and the necessary equipment which reflects the child's specific needs should be prepared.

b. It is important that there is effective communication between the ward and perioperative staff. This will ensure that information regarding delays in the theatre list, prolonged operative procedures and late admissions, for example, reach the relevant staff thus helping to reduce the parental anxiety, ensure pre-medication is given at the appropriate time and prevent children from being starved for longer than necessary.

6. Postoperative and Recovery Room Care

a. Communication is important between the perioperative staff to ensure that all information is given regarding the operative procedures and the necessary postoperative care. In addition, it will be necessary for the recovery staff to be aware of relevant previous history, behavioural or language difficulties and the child's situation.

b. The child should never be left unaccompanied.

c. A full range of paediatric resuscitation equipment must be available at all times.

d. It is essential that qualified recovery staff have a knowledge of the paediatric dosage of medication. Adequate pain control is essential and qualified staff should be available who have the ability to recognise when a child is requiring pain control. Medical staff should be available for the prescribing of adequate analgesia.

e. A non-threatening environment is important. Coloured walls, pictures, posters, toys and patterned coloured curtains are important. The atmosphere should be peaceful and quiet with limited numbers of people and few telephone disturbances.

f. As with all patients in recovery, privacy, dignity and warmth should be maintained with minimal disturbances once the child is settled. Curtains and screens should be available to ensure privacy and dignity.

g. The child should be allowed to find his or her own comfortable position where medically possible.

h. The use of padded trolley sides minimise the risk of injury.

i. The department policy should include an invitation of a parent or carer to the recovery room where possible and parents or carers should be offered the opportunity to accompany the ward nurse to collect their child.

j. All children should be returned to their parents or carers as soon as medically possible.

Principles of Safe Practice in
The Perioperative Environment

Clinical Practice - *Section 3*

Reviewers

Genevieve Rohrlach RGN DipN
Professional Officer
NATN

Chris Fell RGN DipN FETC
Sister & NVQ Co-ordinator
West Suffolk Hospital

Dot Chadwick RGN RM Bsc(Hons) DipN FETC
Clinical Nurse Specialist
Dorset County Hospital

Jacqueline Burbidge RGN
Senior Nurse Practice Development
The Royal Brompton & Harefield NHS Trust

Contributors:

Jenny Asker RGN Dip Research
Clinical Nurse Specialist
United Leeds Teaching Hospitals NHS Trust

Theresa Laurent SEN RGN DipN BANurs
Sister
Leicester General Hospital NHS Trust

Principles of Safe Practice in The Perioperative Environment

Clinical Practice - *Section 3*

PREPARATION OF PERSONNEL

Introduction

Although surgery takes place in numerous types of settings, a patient's surgical outcome is greatly influenced by the creation and maintenance of an aseptic environment. The aim of all perioperative personnel must therefore be to minimise the introduction of microorganisms into the perioperative setting.

Personnel are able to influence the environment by maintaining personal hygiene, wearing theatre attire correctly, reporting potential health problems, monitoring visitors and maintaining a clean environment.

All departments must have written procedures stating the correct preparation of staff entering and leaving all areas of the perioperative environment. All staff must be made aware of these policies and procedures.

Each perioperative environment has established traffic patterns. The design of the department often predetermines these patterns and each area should be clearly indicated.

Unrestricted areas - traffic is not limited.

Semi-restricted areas - traffic is limited to authorised personnel, correctly attired and patients.

Restricted areas - traffic is very limited and personnel must be correctly attired. This includes the operating theatre.

BIBLIOGRAPHY

ACORN 1998 Attire in the Operating Suite. Standards, Guidelines and Policy Statements Australia, ACORN Ltd.

ACORN 1998 Visitors to the Operating Suite. Standards, Guidelines and Policy Statements. Australia, ACORN Ltd.

AORN 1997 Surgical Attire. Standards, Recommended Practices and Guidelines. Denver, AORN Inc.

AORN 1997 Traffic Patterns in the Perioperative Practice Setting. Standards, Recommended Practices and Guidelines. Denver, AORN Inc.

Baumgardner A Maragos C Walz J Larson E 1993 Effects of nail polish on microbial growth of fingernails, dispelling sacred cows. AORN Journal. 58 (1) 84-88

Belkin N 1996 A century after their introduction, are surgical masks necessary. AORN Journal. 64 (4) 602-607

Caudwell M 1998 Sacred Cows and Anti Static Footwear. British Journal of Theatre Nursing. 8 (4) 15-16

Environmental Protection Act 1990

Garner B D 1995 Infection Control. In: Meeker M Rothrock J 1995 Alexander's Care of the Patient in Surgery. (10th Edition) St Louis, Mosby

HSE 1992 The Disposal of Clinical Waste revised

HSE 1996 Protecting your health at work

HSE 1992 Workplace health, safety & welfare - a short guide for managers

McCluskey F 1996 Does wearing a face mask reduce bacterial wound infection? A literature review. British Journal of Theatre Nursing. 6 (5) 18-20, 29

NATN 1997 Universal Precautions and Infection Control in the Perioperative Setting. Harrogate, NATN

NATN 1988 Preparation of Personnel. Principles Of Safe Practice In The Operating Theatre. Harrogate, NATN

NATN 1998 Aseptic Technique. Principles Of Safe Practice In The Perioperative Environment. Harrogate, NATN

NATN 1998 Infection Control in the Perioperative Environment. Principles of Safe Practice in the Perioperative Environment. Harrogate, NATN

NATN 1998 Scrubbing, Gowning and Gloving. Principles Of Safe Practice In The Perioperative Environment. Harrogate, NATN

NATN 1998 The Safeguards for Invasive Procedures : The Management of Risks. Harrogate, NATN

NATN 1998 Universal Precautions. Principles Of Safe Practice In The Perioperative Environment. Harrogate, NATN

NATN 1998 Visitors to the Perioperative Environment. Principles Of Safe Practice In The Perioperative Environment. Harrogate, NATN

NHS Estates 1991 Health Building Notes 26 Operating Department. London, HMSO

NHS Estates 1994 A Strategic to Clinical Waste Management

Norman A 1995 A comparison of face masks and visors for the scrub team. British Journal of Theatre Nursing. 5 (2) 10-13

Riley R 1997 The wearing of surgical masks: striking a balance. ACORN Journal. 10 (1) 31-34

Taylor M Campbell C 1998 Surgical Practice. In: Clarke C Jones J Brigden's Operating Department Practice. Edinburgh, Churchill Livingstone

Thomas J A Fligelstone L J Jerwood T E Rees R W M 1993 Theatre Footwear: A Health Hazard? British Journal of Theatre Nursing. 3 (7) 5-9

Wicker C P 1997 Sacred cows and sound practice. British Journal of Theatre Nursing. 7 (7) 31-34

Recommendations for Inclusion in Local Policy

1. Changing Areas

i. Adequate, suitable and secure storage facilities should be available for staff clothing and for theatre attire. These changing facilities should be readily accessible but ensure privacy for the user.

ii. It is recommended that there is adequate provision for disposal of used theatre clothing. Linen and rubbish bags should be used and disposed of in accordance with local policy.

iii. It is essential that an adequate supply of clean theatre clothes are available at all times and that this clothing is stored in a clean, dry condition.

2. Theatre Attire

Theatre attire, which may include scrub clothes, hair covering, masks, eye-wear, plastic aprons and other barriers, are worn to provide protection from contamination for both patients and staff.

i. All personnel who enter the semi-restricted and restricted areas of the perioperative environment should be in clean freshly laundered theatre attire.

ii. Clothing should be made of a close woven coloured material that is easily washed at high temperatures, lint free, cool, comfortable, in good repair and give a professional appearance.

iii. Trouser suits, as opposed to dresses, are deemed micro-biologically superior. Loose, flapping clothing are sources of possible contamination as personnel move, and should be avoided.

iv. Theatre attire should be changed when it becomes soiled or wet.

v. Clean, lint free surgical hats or hoods that completely cover all head and facial hair should be provided. Double woven disposal paper hats are recommended.

vi. Footwear should provide support and protection for the feet, be easy to clean and only worn within the designated areas.

vii. Disposable high filtration face masks should be provided near the restricted areas. They must be worn in accordance with local policy, completely covering nose and mouth and secured by tapes. Masks should not be handled except when being put on and taken off. They should only be handled by the tapes and discarded into the appropriate receptacles on removal. Masks should be changed when soiled and every two hours when possible. They should be removed completed when leaving the restricted areas.

Current research questions the need to wear masks during surgical procedures. In some instances it may only be necessary for personnel within the immediate vicinity of the operative site to wear masks, and then mostly for occupational health and safety reasons. Healthy persons undergoing elective surgery are at a minimal risk of contracting wound infections. In contrast, persons who are immunosuppressed, have malignancies, diabetes, are elderly or chronically ill or undergoing prosthetic implants are at great risk of contracting wound infection and need every possible precaution to be taken. Literature suggests that emphasis should be placed on enforcing the basic elements of perioperative practice and aseptic technique rather than relying on masks to prevent wound infections. The principles of universal blood and body substance isolation precautions must also be considered when writing policies on the wearing of masks.

3. Preparation of Personnel

All personnel who work within the perioperative setting are responsible for reporting instances of ill health and infection to a senior member of staff before they enter the perioperative environment. Reference to the occupational health department should be made as necessary.

a. Perioperative Personnel

i. It is essential that all staff receive instruction as to the correct manner of dress within the operating department, including information about the need for strict personal hygiene and good health and the implications of these to patient care.

ii. It is recommended that all staff change in the following manner: all outer clothes and jewellery should be removed or confined within theatre attire. Hands should be washed, a surgical hat or hood is placed over the hair ensuring all is covered. Freshly laundered theatre clothing is chosen, clean footwear is put on, hands are washed again once changing procedure is complete.

iii. Fingernails should be kept short, clean and free of nail polish and artificial nails.

iv. It is essential that personnel are able to shower and change theatre attire should they become contaminated.

v. At the end of a span of duty theatre attire should be discarded in accordance with local policy. Home laundering is not recommended as it is not conducive with infection control protocols.

vi. Surgical attire should not be worn outside the perioperative environment. All personnel should change into outer clothes when leaving the perioperative environment, and don a new set of theatre attire on their return.

vii. If it is not feasible to follow the above practice, cover apparel may be worn when leaving the perioperative environment. A clean single use gown or coat, completely secured by ties or button fasteners, should be worn one time and discarded appropriately. The use of cover apparel should be determined by the individual practice setting.

viii. Protective attire should be provided and worn in accordance with occupational health and safety standards. Employees should remember that they have a responsibility to co-operate with any measures that their employer may take to protect their health in the workplace.

b. **Visitors to Perioperative Environment**

More comprehensive recommendations regarding visitors in the perioperative environment can be found in this document in 'Visitors to the Perioperative Environment'. In the interest of good perioperative practice and for patient confidentiality and dignity, visitors to the perioperative environment should be kept to a minimum and only be admitted if they have obtained permission from the appropriate person(s) for bona-fide supportive or educational reasons.

i. There must be a local policy regarding visitors to the perioperative environment and unauthorised personnel should not enter.

ii. Visitors must be introduced to the designated senior member of staff and be issued with suitable identification before entering the area.

iii. Visitors should enter by the designed route and be chaperoned at all times.

iv. Visitors under the age of 18 years should be actively discouraged.

v. It is essential that personnel intending to observe within the perioperative environment follow the recommendations referred to in 'Preparation of Personnel', within this section.

vi. It is essential that all visitors to the perioperative environment are made aware that all procedures within this environment are confidential in nature and that any information, discussions, technical details or documentation data must be treated in confidence.

Principles of Safe Practice in The Perioperative Environment

Clinical Practice - *Section 3*

VISITORS TO THE PERIOPERATIVE ENVIRONMENT

Introduction

Visitors approach the perioperative environment for various reasons and there is often pressure for access to be given. It must be remembered that the paramount aim of perioperative practice is **patient care** and all visitors must accept this as the priority.

Patients have the right to confidentiality unless they have consented to have information divulged. Patients have the **right to refuse** the presence of visitors during their perioperative phase. Only visitors who have obtained permission for definite supportive and/or educational reasons should be allowed in the operating department during a patient's perioperative phase. The number of visitors permitted to the perioperative environment should be kept to a minimum.

BIBLIOGRAPHY

ACORN 1998 Visitors to the Operating Suite. Standards, Guidelines and Policy Statements, Australia, ACORN Ltd.

Data Protection Act 1984

NATN 1988 Visitors to the Operating Department. Principles Of Safe Practice In The Operating Theatre. Harrogate, NATN

NATN 1996 Nursing the Paediatric Patient in the Adult Perioperative Environment. Harrogate, NATN

NATN 1997 Universal Precautions and Infection Control in the Perioperative Setting. Harrogate, NATN

NATN 1998 Aseptic Technique. Principles Of Safe Practice In The Perioperative Environment. Harrogate, NATN

NATN 1998 Preparation of Personnel. Principles Of Safe Practice In The Perioperative Environment. Harrogate, NATN

NATN 1998 Universal Precautions. Principles Of Safe Practice In The Perioperative Environment. Harrogate, NATN

NAWCH 1990 Reducing the Stress of Operation Day: Parent Involvement, London, NAWCH

O'Neill S 1992 Children in Recovery. Nursing Times. 88 (41) 68-70

Smith B 1997 Attendance of company representatives in the operating theatre. British Journal of Theatre Nursing. 7 (1) 40

Tunner P 1997 Establishing a protocol for parental presence in recovery. British Journal of Nursing. 6 (14) 794-799

UKCC 1992 Code of Professional Conduct. (third edition) London, UKCC

Recommendations for Inclusion in Local Policy

1. General Considerations

i. It is essential that each department has a written policy stating the correct protocol for visitors to the environment and that all staff are aware of the policy.

ii. It is essential that all visitors gain permission to enter the perioperative environment prior to their visit, and on arrival, must report their presence to the appointed person.

iii. It is essential that there is a control mechanism for authorisation of people visiting the perioperative environment, which should include documentation of their arrival and departure in a specific register.

iv. It is essential that all visitors are provided with the necessary theatre attire and have an understanding of how it is worn. Visitors should be clearly identified as such, i.e. with a visitor identity badge.

v. It is essential that visitors are made aware that all procedures within the perioperative environment are confidential in nature and that any information, discussions, technical details or documentation data must be treated in confidence.

vi. All visitors should be made aware of perioperative etiquette and if they are observing clinical procedures they should be introduced to the staff in the area.

vii. It is essential that visitors are chaperoned **at all times** during their stay in the perioperative environment.

viii. Visitors must understand the procedure should they feel faint or unwell during their stay.

ix. It is essential that medical, nursing and technical personnel, who are not designated employees of the hospital, but wish to participate during their visit, have their professional qualification(s) and health status endorsed prior to admission.

2. Special consideration

a. Photography/Video

i. It is essential that any visitor wishing to use photographic equipment during their visit to the perioperative environment applies for the necessary permission.

ii It should be remembered that it is necessary to gain consent from patients before photographs are taken.

iii. Any photographs taken of patients are the copyright of the Secretary of State for Health, and may only be used subsequently if further permission is gained from the patient.

iv When outside agencies have been given permission to film or photograph within the perioperative environment, it is recommended that staff are reminded of their role in patient advocacy and standards of professional conduct.

v. Media personnel should not be permitted into the perioperative environment without permission from the hospital's administration.

b. Relatives, Friends and Staff accompany patients.

It is recommended that patients with special needs or requirements are accompanied into the perioperative environment by a support person. The following are examples of special needs and requirements.

i.   Children who are undergoing surgery may be accompanied to the anaesthetic room by a parent or carer or at least by a ward nurse who is familiar to the child. It is important however, to respect the wishes of the parent or carer. Local policies should reflect a multidisciplinary agreed protocol that supports this initiative.

ii. Parents or carers should be considered a useful asset in the recovery area, and their presence should be encouraged.

iii. Women taken to theatre for caesarean section may be accompanied in the theatre by their partners, if the woman so wishes. The partner should be appropriately prepared in the protocols to be observed during the perioperative phase.

iv. Patients with language problems may be accompanied to theatre by a relative or friend who can interpret for them, or by an interpreter.

v.   Confused patients may be accompanied by someone they know.

vi. Psychiatric patients may be accompanied by an RMN.

It is recommended that a designed waiting area be provided for relatives and friends that it is situated away from the perioperative environment.

c. **Security of Persons**

There are certain instances when patients have to be accompanied by an officer e.g. royalty and patients under police custody. The attendance of these officers has to be given special consideration.

d. **Company Representatives**

The attendance of company representatives in the perioperative environment is sometimes requested. It should be remembered that demonstrations of new technology should take place in a workshop or laboratory setting, and perioperative staff should be familiar with the technology prior to direct patient use.

There are implications for the company representative, medical staff and the hospital that must be addressed prior to admission being granted. These implications include patient consent, medical indemnity, confidentiality, health screening and the role of the representative within the perioperative environment.

Principles of Safe Practice in The Perioperative Environment

Clinical Practice - *Section 3*

CARE AND HANDLING OF SPECIMENS

Introduction

In the operating theatre specimens are regularly taken during surgical procedures. It is essential that every specimen reaches the pathology, bacteriology, histology or cytology department without undue delay and in optimum condition.

Specimen pathophysiology is important for determining subsequent treatment of the patient and the care and handling is a crucial step in the investigations. It is therefore recommended that perioperative staff are aware of the procedures involved in the care of specimens, including correct documentation, safe handling and the appropriate despatch of specimens. Further information is available from the local hospital Pathology Services Handbook.

BIBLIOGRAPHY

Anthony P MacSweer R 1997 Recent Advances in Histopathology. London, Churchill Livingstone

Control of Substances Hazardous to Health Regulations 1988

DHSS 1991 Codes of Practice for the Prevention of Infection in Clinical Laboratories and Post Mortem Rooms

Fabian D 1991 Handling Laboratory Specimens in a Medical Office, Professional Medical Assistant. 24 (1) 6-7

Human Tissue Act 1961

NATN 1988 Care and Handling of Specimens. Principles Of Safe Practice In The Operating Theatre. Harrogate, NATN

NATN 1997 Universal Precautions and Infection Control in the perioperative setting. Harrogate, NATN

NATN 1998 Universal Precautions. Principles Of Safe Practice In The Perioperative Environment. Harrogate, NATN

NATN 1998 Infection Control. Principles Of Safe Practice In The Perioperative Environment. Harrogate, NATN

Pierson M A 1995 Patient and Environmental Safety. In: Meeker M H Rothrock J C 1995 Alexander's Care of the Patient in Surgery. (10th Edition) St Louis, Mosby

NHS Management Executive 1991 Disposal of Foetal Tissue. HSG (91) 19, November. London, DOH

Recommendations for Inclusion in Local Policy

1. Safe Handling and Dispatch of Specimens

a. It is essential that the scrub person checks with the surgeon the following details:

    i. the nature of the specimen

    ii. the site from which the specimen was taken

b. It is recommended that care is taken in selecting an appropriate specimen container. The container should be large enough to ensure that the specimen floats freely, is completely covered by appropriate fixative and sealed for transportation.

c. It is essential that the circulating person follows universal blood and body substance isolation precautions when placing the specimen in the container. Precautions also need to be taken to prevent any contamination of the outside of the specimen container.

d. All staff should adhere to COSHH regulations and local policies for treatment in respect of splash injuries from specimen fixative or body fluids.

e. All specimens for bacteriology should be placed in a specified biohazard bag and sealed before dispatch.

f. Universal blood and body substance isolation precautions should always be used when handling specimens as all specimens are considered a potential source of infection.

2. Documentation

a. Once the specimen has been placed into the container it is essential that a member of the perioperative team labels the specimen container immediately. The label must NOT be placed on the lid of the container, as this could cause potential confusion over the specimens.

b. After checking with the patient's notes, the details on the label and the request form should include:

    i. The patient's full name,

    ii. The patient's identification number,

    iii. Date of birth,

    iv. Ward, hospital, theatre,

    v. Details of the nature of the specimen,

    vi. Date/time specimen was taken,

    vii. Details of the nature of fixative.

c. The information on the investigation request form must correspond with the details on the specimen container and the patient's notes.

d. It is the responsibility of the medical officer to sign the request form and state what particular investigations are required.

f. It is extremely important that all information is accurate and checked before the specimen leaves the operating theatre. The specimen must be accompanied by the documentation.

g. It is recommended that a signed record is kept of all specimens dispatched from the operating theatre.

3. Specimens Requiring Special Consideration

a. Frozen Sections

    i. It is the responsibility of the medical staff to give notification to the histology department of specimens requiring frozen section and to complete the investigation request form prior to starting the operation.

ii. Specimens for frozen section are placed in dry containers, labelled as stated (2,b) and must be despatched immediately to the appropriate department.

b. **Foreign Bodies**

i. Must be clearly labelled and retained for inspection.

ii. Forensic specimens must be saved in accordance with the Human Tissue Act 1961 and local policies, ensuring that there is total traceability of the specimen at all times until it reaches its destination.

c. **Orthopaedic Implants**

When orthopaedic implants are to be removed, care should be taken to ascertain:

i. Whether the implant is to be sent for bacteriology, pathological, metallurgical or mechanical examination.

ii. The legal ownership of the implant before any destructive testing is carried out.

d. **Retained Products of Conception**

i. Account is taken of any personal wishes expressed in respect of a foetus or foetal tissue.

ii. Laboratory staff are informed of any personal wishes expressed if a foetus or foetal tissue needs to be sent for pathological examination.

iii. Foetal tissue is treated in accordance with Health Service Guidelines. HSG (91) 19. (NHS Management Executive 1991).

Principles of Safe Practice in The Perioperative Environment

Clinical Practice - *Section 3*

SCRUBBING, GOWNING AND GLOVING

Introduction

The techniques employed by perioperative personnel when preparing themselves to take part in sterile procedures can be varied. However, the fundamental principles of aseptic technique **must** be adhered to when scrubbing, gowning and gloving prior to surgical intervention.

It is necessary for each department to have a standardised procedure and that the method used is practised to a high level of competence.

The following sets out the principles of safe practice in the perioperative environment and offer recommendations for each technique. These recommendations should be read in conjunction with appropriate sections of this document.

BIBLIOGRAPHY

ACORN 1998 Surgical Scrubbing, Gowning and Gloving. Standards, Guidelines and Policy Statements. Australia, ACORN Ltd.

AORN 1997 Hands Scrubs, Surgical. Standards Recommended Practices and Guidelines. Denver, AORN Inc.

Baumgardner C Maragos C Walz J Larson E 1993 Effects of nail polish on microbial growth of fingernails. AORN Journal. 58 (1) 84-88

Eccleston S B 1992 Gloving, Clinical Question Demands Further Research, AORN Journal. 56 (2) 265-269

Fay M 1996 Latex Sensitization. South African Theatre Sisters Journal. 21 (1) 27-34

French G L 1994 Surgical scrub and skin preparation. Surgery Journal. 12 (2) 42-43

Garner B D 1995 Infection Control. In: Meeker M H Rothrock J C 1995 Alexander's Care of the Patient in Surgery. Mosby, St Louis

ICNA 1997 Guidelines for Hand Hygiene. Derbyshire, Deb Ltd.

MDA 1996 Latex sensitisation in the health care setting. BD9601. London, HMSO

NATN 1997 Universal Precautions and Infection Control in the perioperative setting. Harrogate, NATN

NATN 1998 Aseptic Technique. Principles Of Safe Practice In The Perioperative Environment. Harrogate, NATN

NATN 1998 Infection Control. Principles Of Safe Practice In The Perioperative Environment. Harrogate, NATN

NATN 1998 Preparation of Personnel. Principles Of Safe Practice In The Perioperative Environment. Harrogate, NATN

NATN 1998 Safeguards for Invasive Procedures The Management of Risks Harrogate, NATN

NATN 1988 Scrubbing, Gowning and Gloving. Principles Of Safe Practice In The Operating Theatre. Harrogate, NATN

NATN 1998 The Count. Principles Of Safe Practice In The Perioperative Environment. Harrogate, NATN

NATN 1998 Trolley Preparation for Surgical Intervention. Principles Of Safe Practice In The Perioperative Environment. Harrogate, NATN

NATN 1998 Universal Precautions. Principles Of Safe Practice In The Perioperative Environment. Harrogate, NATN

NATN 1998 Use and Handling of Instruments. Principles Of Safe Practice In The Perioperative Environment. Harrogate, NATN

NHS Estates 1991 Health Building Notes 26 Operating Department. London, HMSO

Nightingale K 1996 Ban Glove Powder - An International Symposium. British Journal of Theatre Nursing. 6 (5) 15-16

Poole C J M 1997 Hazards of powdered surgical gloves. The Lancet. 350:9083 973-974

Ross C 1994 What cost ritual? British Journal of Theatre Nursing. 4 (4) 11-14

Shoup A J 1997 Guidelines for the management of latex allergies and safe use of latex in perioperative practice settings, AORN Journal. 66 (4) 726-730

Thomson C M 1996 The Potential Risks of Latex. British Journal of Theatre Nursing. 6 (5) 12-14

Taylor M Campbell C 1998 Surgical Practice. In: Clarke P Jones J Brigden's Operating Department Practice Edinburgh, Churchill Livingstone

Recommendations for Inclusion in Local Policy

The five main areas for consideration are:

1. Facilities
2. Scrubbing procedures
3. Gowning
4. Gloving
5. Post procedure protocol

1. Facilities

i. It is recommended that the "scrub area" is separate from the operating theatre. There should be two entrances - one from the access corridor with a door barrier and the other from the theatre itself with independent access. The size of the room should facilitate free movement of people.

ii. The sink and furniture should be at a height to facilitate hand and arm washing. The design and drainage should ensure that the floor does not become wet during washing procedures. Foot pedals and/or elbow adjustments should be provided to operate taps and dispense scrub solution. Provision of hot and cold water is essential and water should flow at a steady rate. The maintenance of these facilities should be included in a planned preventative maintenance programme.

iii. As wet floors are a potential safety risk, it is important that floor surfaces should be anti-slip.

iv. A shelf or other work surface should be provided on which to open gown packs. This should be at a height to facilitate gowning and gloving, and be wide enough to allow gown packs to be opened fully.

v. Storage facilities for all necessary sterile equipment should be available and located away from the sterile field. Where sterile equipment is stored in the scrub area, it should be situated away from the sink in order to prevent water contamination.

vi. Adequate disposal bins for used brushes and waste paper should be provided.

vii. The scrub area should be kept adequately stocked with necessary equipment. Careful consideration should be paid to the number of sterile gowns required to be stored in the scrub area ensuring adequate stock rotation.

viii. Some microbiocidal scrub preparations have caused problems for individual perioperative staff when allergic reactions have developed. Alternative scrub solutions should be provided. Brushes may be provided for use on nails only.

2. Scrubbing

a. The aim of the surgical scrub is to effectively reduce the number of microorganisms on the skin by mechanical washing. All staff should be in the appropriate theatre attire before beginning a surgical scrub.

This includes the following:

i. Theatre attire secured, i.e. top tucked into trousers and sleeves rolled to well above elbow.

ii. Freshly donned face mask, correctly positioned over the nose and mouth and fitted comfortably.

iii. All hair covered under a surgical hat.

iv. Clean hands and nails; nails short and free of nail polish or artificial nails. Although research has not found a relationship between increased microbial growth and freshly applied polish on fingernails there is a suggestion that personnel may be more concerned with the state of their nails than with performing the surgical scrub to an appropriate standard.

vi. Being free from jewellery. Microorganisms may be harboured under jewellery and/or cause allergic skin reactions resulting from accumulated scrub agents.

vii. Protective eye wear, spectacles and Microscopic glasses   positioned and secured.

viii. Intact skin on hands and arms.

ix. Protective clothing (lead or plastic aprons) donned and comfortable.

b. In order to minimise contamination during the scrubbing procedure, staff should ensure at all times:

i. The water is of a comfortable temperature and steady flow.

ii. The hands are above the level of the elbows.

iii. That care should be taken not to splash theatre clothing.

iv. That movements are steady.

v. That rinsing is performed from fingertips to elbows, using water flow and not hands. Vigorous shaking to dispel water from hands and arms is unacceptable.

c. The practitioner should be aware that the purpose of the scrub procedure is to attack the transient and resident microorganisms on the hands and arms. This can only be successful if the scrub solution stays in contact with the skin. Approximately 5 mls of scrub solution should be dispensed at each application and this should be worked into the hands and arms before washing off.

Dispensing copious amounts of scrub solution followed by quick application and rinsing, is neither efficient in technique nor cost effective.

d. The following scrub procedure identifies three stages which are effective for preoperative hand disinfection. The first wash should encompass the hands and arms to the elbows. Subsequent washes should not reach as far as the elbows as this will compromise the effectiveness of the scrubbing technique, two thirds of the forearm is considered an adequate level.

e. The brush should be used for the first scrub of the operating session only and always follows the first wash of the procedure. Only the nails are to be brushed. Brushing other areas of the hands and arms has been shown to be detrimental to the skin surface causing abrasions. This principle applies also to pre-packed impregnated sterile brushes.

f. It is recommended that two sterile disposable paper towels are used for drying the hands and arms. Rubbing the skin in order to dry it, will disturb skin cells. The skin should be blotted dry with the towels.

g. Adhering to the principle that it is important to work from fingertips to elbows:

   i. The hand is dried first.

   ii. A corkscrew movement should be used to blot the arm dry from the hand to the elbow. The towel should be folded so that the drying hand is protected from contact with the arms.

   iii. The towel is discarded immediately.

   iv. The process is repeated for the other arm.

3. Gowning Procedure

a. Various styles of gowns are available, made from variety of fabrics and in several styles.

   Whichever style is chosen, all staff should be aware of :

   i. The specification of the gown.

   ii. How it is packed and presented.

   iii. How it is donned.

   iv. Once donned, what area of sterility it affords the wearer.

   It is recommended that gowns should be made from a non permeable material and should be "wrap around" in style.

b. All gowns should be presented in a good state of repair and any gown found not to

have been processed to a high standard should be discarded.

It is essential that a variety of sizes are available to staff and that staff discard any gown that is too small and therefore unsafe for their use.

c. As the gown is donned:

   i. The practitioner must ensure that they touch the inside of the gown only and that both arms are inserted into the sleeves of the gown together.

   ii. The circulating person should assist the scrubbed person by securing the gown's back ties.

4. Gloving Procedures

a. The closed gloving is the method of choice in most operating departments. However, there is a place for the open method. The effectiveness of either method is in the way in which they are performed, poor technique will compromise sterility whichever method is chosen.

b. Alternative gloves should be made available for perioperative personnel who are sensitive to latex. All starch powdered latex gloves should be removed from the environment.

c. When gloves require changing intra-operatively because of puncture or inadvertent contamination, the preferred method is for one member of the sterile team to glove the other. However, if this is not possible, the contaminated glove should be removed in such a way as to avoid further contamination and can be changed by either the open or closed gloving method.

5. Post Procedure Protocol

a. Once all procedures have been completed, it is essential that the practitioner understands that their area of sterility is;

   i. From fingertips to elbows.

   ii. Below nipple line to waist level.

b. The hands must be kept at or above waist level at all times

c. When not involved in a sterile procedure the scrubbed person should stand with their hands within the area of sterility, palms together.

d. At the end of the sterile procedure, the practitioner should remove first the gown over gloved hands and then the gloves, disposing of them in accordance with the local policy. Hands should then be washed and dried.

Principles of Safe Practice in The Perioperative Environment

Clinical Practice - *Section 3*

THE COUNT

(SWABS, INSTRUMENTS AND NEEDLES)

Introduction

The overriding principle for the count is that all swabs, instruments and sharps must be accounted for, at all times during an invasive surgical procedure, to prevent foreign body retention and subsequent injury to the patient.

Although it is the responsibility of the user to return all items, it is recognised as 'custom and practice' that the scrub person implements the checking procedure in order to be able to state categorically that all items have been returned.

The count must be audible to those counting and be conducted by two members of staff, one of whom MUST be an appropriately qualified member of the perioperative team (i.e. a registered nurse or a qualified ODA or ODP Level 3).

A count must be undertaken for all procedures in which the likelihood exists that swabs, instruments and/or sharps could be retained.

Countable items may include, but are not limited to:

X-ray detectable gauze swabs, packs, lahey swabs (peanuts), gauze strips, neuro patties, needles, instruments, blades, local infiltration needles, tapes, slings, bulldogs.

BIBLIOGRAPHY

ACORN 1998 Counting of Accountable Items. Standards, Guidelines and Policy Statements. Australia, ACORN Ltd.

AORN 1997 Sponge, Sharp and Instrument Counts. Standards, Recommended Practices and Guidelines. Denver, AORN Inc.

Bynom S 1998 Reflection - a lost swab. British Journal of Theatre Nursing. 8 (5) 15-18

Fish J 1992 An alternative to swab racks. Nursing Standard. 7 (3) 55-56

Fulbrook S 1995 Duty of Care. British Journal of Theatre Nursing. 5 (5) 18-19

Lamb A 1992 The Swab Rack - an outdated ritual. British Journal of Theatre Nursing. 2 (2) 14-17

Langslow A 1992 Relying on the count. The Australian Nurses Journal. 21 (11) 31-32

Langslow A 1992 More on foreign bodies. The Australian Nurses Journal. 22 (1) 30-31

MDA 1998 Reporting adverse incidents relating to medical devices.

SN 9801

Murphy E K 1991 Liability for inaccurate counts. AORN Journal. 53 (1) 157-161

NATN 1997 Universal Precautions and Infection Control in the Perioperative Setting. Harrogate, NATN

NATN 1998 Infection Control. Principles Of Safe Practice In The Perioperative Environment. Harrogate, NATN

NATN 1998 Safeguards for Invasive Procedures : The Management of Risks. Harrogate, NATN

NATN 1988 The Count. Principles Of Safe Practice In The Operating Theatre. Harrogate, NATN

NATN 1998 Universal Precautions. Principles Of Safe Practice In The Perioperative Environment. Harrogate, NATN

NATN 1998 Use and Handling of Instruments. Principles Of Safe Practice In The Perioperative Environment. Harrogate, NATN

Olsen C 1995 Sutures, Needles, and Instruments. In: Meeker M H 1995 Alexander's Care of the Patient in Surgery. (10th Edition) Mosby, St Louis

Taylor M Campbell C 1998 Surgical Practice In: Clarke P Jones J (Eds) Brigdens. Operating Department Practice. Edinburgh, Churchill Livingstone

Tingle J 1997 Legal problems in the operating theatre: learning from mistakes. British Journal of Nursing. 6 (15) 889-891

UKCC 1992 Code of Professional Conduct. (3rd Edition) London, UKCC

Recommendations for Inclusion in Local Policy

The main areas for consideration are:

1. Education/Training
2. Packaging
3. Responsibility for counts
4. Checking Procedure
5. Counting Techniques
6. Count Discrepancy

1. Education/Training

a. Where a hospital runs a perioperative course the post basic nursing student or trainee ODP should have supernumerary status until they have been deemed competent for this skill.

b. An introduction to the local policy **must** be included in all new staff's orientation programme.

2. Packaging

a. All swabs, including lahey swabs (peanuts), neuro patties and packs, that are used during invasive procedures must have an x-ray detectable marker fixed securely across the width of the swab.

b. All swabs and packs must be packed in bundles of five (5) and be of a uniform size and weight. Any package containing fewer or more than five should be removed from the procedure area immediately. Checks should be made based on multiples of five.

3. Responsibility for counts

a. Each count must be performed by two members of staff, one of whom **must** be a qualified perioperative practitioner (i.e. not a learner). The staff involved in the counting procedure must be able to recognise and identify the equipment in use.

b. The same two perioperative personnel should perform all the counts that are done during the surgical procedure.

   i. Should it be necessary to replace either person during the procedure, a complete count should be performed, recorded and signed by the incoming and outgoing practitioners.

   ii. Should it be necessary to replace either person temporarily, the relieving practitioner should follow the standard procedure and note and sign any additions on the intraoperative record.

  iii. The name of the replacement or relieving practitioner must be recorded on the intraoperative record.

c. Items which are to remain in the patient by intention (for example packing gauze, drain tubes, catheters) must be recorded in the intraoperative record. When a countable item is **deliberately** left in a patient, this must be recorded on the intraoperative form/theatre register/patient's notes. Its removal must also be recorded.

d. All items must remain in the operating theatre until the procedure has been completed and all counts have been performed.

e. Swabs that are used as surface dressing must not be x-ray detectable. These swabs should only be opened at skin closure.

4. Checking Procedure

a. A swab, instrument and needle count should be performed for all surgical procedures and recorded immediately. This record should be retained in the patient's notes.

b. Provision should be made in the theatre for a dry wipe count board, which is pre-printed and states all relevant items used. This board should be permanently fixed to the theatre wall and be at a height and in a position that facilitates access and visibility during the procedure.

c. The initial count must be performed immediately prior to the commencement of surgery.

d. Items added during the procedure must be counted and recorded. There should be a

local system of accounting for instruments that are used during the procedure.

e. At all times during a surgical procedure the scrub person must be aware of the location of all equipment. Neatness in approach should be encouraged to ensure that only necessary equipment is in use at any given time.

f. If a blade, needle or instrument breaks during use, the scrub person should ensure that all pieces have been returned and are accounted for. Any instrument found to be damaged will compromise patient safety and therefore must be immediately taken out of use and labelled for repair. It may be necessary to inform the Supplies Department, the Manufactures and/or DOH if an obvious fault is found with equipment. If appropriate, the DOH will issue a Hazard Warning or Safety Bulletin.

g. A count should be performed at the commencement of the closure of any cavity and the final count at the commencement of skin closure. Instruments and items with screws and/or removable parts should also be included in the count. The surgical team must allow time for these counts to be undertaken without pressure.

h. On completion of the final count a verbal statement should be made by the scrub person to the effect that all equipment is accounted for and verbal acknowledgement should be received from the surgeon in order to alleviate any misunderstanding.

i. At the end of the surgical procedure the circulating and scrub persons must record that satisfactory checks have taken in the relevant documentation. This should include the theatre records and the patient's notes.

5. Checking Techniques

a. Both practitioners must count aloud and items should be completely separated during the checking procedure.

b. The integrity of the x-ray detectable markers in swabs, packs, peanuts etc. must be checked during the count.

c. At the initial count, and when added during the procedure, swabs and packs should be counted into separate groups of five. These should not be added to those already counted until verification of the number in the packet. The additions should be in multiples of five.

d. In the event of an incorrect number of swabs or packs (i.e. not five) the entire packet must be removed from the procedure area.

e. If any interruption occurs during the counting procedure, the count should be recommenced.

f. Swabs and packs should be counted off the sterile field. The technique used should be safe and incorporate infection control measure in conjunction with Universal Precautions. All items should be fully opened and counted in multiples of five before, **and** as they are placed into a plastic bag. The bag should be sealed and the number of contents recorded on the bag. The items in the sealed bags should be counted at closure counts according to the number on the bag. If there is a discrepancy in the closure counts, all bags should be opened and their contents recounted. Swab racks must not be used.

g. Items should not be cut or altered unless specifically intended for the purpose. If alterations of any item is requested by the person performing the procedure this **must** be documented and included in the count.

6. Count Discrepancy

a. If any discrepancy in the count is identified, the surgeon must be informed immediately and a thorough search implemented at once.

b. If a thorough search does not locate the item, an x-ray should be taken before the patient leaves the operating theatre.

c. Missing micro items, (for example: needles which **cannot** be detected on x-ray) should be recorded on the intraoperative record and theatre register. X-ray should be performed at the discretion of the surgeon.

d. All missing items must be documented. Formal incident procedures must be followed in accordance with local policy. The discrepancy and subsequent action must be reported to the appropriate personnel and a record must be made.

Principles of Safe Practice in The Perioperative Environment

Clinical Practice - *Section 3*

TROLLEY PREPARATION FOR SURGICAL INTERVENTION

Introduction

The type of surgery being performed may influence the type of instrument trolley that is used. All trolleys should adhere to the Medical Devices Directive 93/42 and be stable and robust enough for the intended job. The design choice of the instrument trolley will need to take into account ease of movement, height and ease of cleaning in accordance with local infection control policies. They should be included in a planned prevention maintenance programme. Particular attention to wheel mechanisms is required in order to allow free and smooth movement. The trolleys, mayo stands and bowl stands should be made of aluminium, stainless steel or mild steel covered in nylon. All trolleys should be free of abrasions and be in good working order.

The preparation of sterile instrument trolleys for surgical intervention is a skilled and precise procedure that requires adherence to a strict aseptic technique throughout.

BIBLIOGRAPHY

Environment Protection Act 1990.

Johnson M 1994 Planning Operating Departments. Who does it? British Journal Theatre Nurses. 4 (7) 13

MDA 1998 All class 1 items (those items involved with patient contact) should have EC. 'CE' markings as of June 1998.

NATN 1997 Universal precautions and infection control in the perioperative setting. Harrogate, NATN

NATN 1998 Aseptic Technique, Principles Of Safe Practice In The Perioperative Environment. Harrogate, NATN

NATN 1998 Infection Control. Principles Of Safe Practice In The Perioperative Environment. Harrogate, NATN

NATN 1988 Trolley preparation for surgical intervention. Principles Of Safe Practice In The Operatng Theatre. Harrogate, NATN

NHS Estates 1991 Health Building Notes 26 Operating Department. London, HMSO

NHS Estates 1994 A Strategic Guide to Clinical Waste

Rawlinson C 1985 Appraisal of theatre provision in a district general hospital: a case study. Medical Architectural Research Unit

Vincent S 1998 Surgical Intervention, Facilities for the year 2010 and beyond. British Journal of Theatre Nursing. 7 (10) 12-15

Recommendations for Inclusion in Local Policy

General Considerations

1. The instruments must be prepared immediately prior to each individual surgical intervention in accordance with the planned operative procedure and individual patient needs.

2. A designated area, which affords sufficient space to open packs and maintain a sterile field, should be identified for this procedure. Furthermore, there should be minimal movement of personnel within this area during preparation of the trolley.

3. All equipment for the surgical procedure must be gathered in advance and all packs to be used must be checked for sterility and damage.

4. Two members of staff are required for the preparation of sterile trolleys. It is essential that one of these members are scrubbed, gowned and gloved and follow the principles of aseptic technique. All trolleys should be covered with at least two layers of sterile drapes. The drapes should be of a recommended material large enough to cover the horizontal plane of the trolley and enough vertical plane to avoid contamination. Sterile equipment must be presented to the person from the edge of the sterile field and received in such a way as to prevent glove contamination on the unsterile wraps. The trolley should be considered sterile on the horizontal plane only. Once prepared the trolley must be attended at all times.

5. It is recommended that there should be a locally agreed method of laying out sterile instrument trolleys. All staff should adhere to this method in order to facilitate continuity of patient care and safety in the event of a sudden change of scrub person during the operative procedure.

6. Trolleys should be placed correctly around or over the patient depending on the planned operative procedure. Care must be taken to ensure that there is no undue pressure placed on any part of the patient's body or limbs.

7. All instruments must be returned to the surface of the instrument trolley in order to prevent injury to the patient.

8. Any break in aseptic technique must be acted on immediately. Contaminated equipment must be removed from the sterile field using a suitable instrument to prevent compromising sterility of the procedure. Re-gloving and re-draping should be carried out where appropriate.

9. The disposal of all equipment, drapes and sharps must be carried out in accordance with local and national guidelines. The scrub person should be considered the person of choice to dispose of all contaminated materials whilst still gowned and gloved.

Principles of Safe Practice in The Perioperative Environment

Clinical Practice - *Section 3*

ASEPTIC TECHNIQUE

Introduction

The outcome of a patient's surgical experience is influenced by the knowledge and application of aseptic technique by the perioperative staff. All persons involved in the preparation and performance of surgical procedures are responsible for providing a safe environment for the patient. This is best achieved by maintaining asepsis and limiting the risk of contamination.

Measures to prevent surgical wound infection include provision of supplies and equipment which are free of microbial contamination at the time of use. Sterilisation provides the highest level of assurance that an object is void of viable microbes. Disinfection reduces the risk of microbial contamination but without the same level of assurance.

The basic principles of aseptic technique prevent contamination of the open wound, isolate the operative site from the surrounding unsterile physical environment and create and maintain a sterile field so that surgery can be performed safely.

This principle should be used in conjunction with the recommendations outlined within this document.

BIBLIOGRAPHY

ACORN 1998 Aseptic Technique in the Operating Suite. Standards, Guidelines and Policy Statements. Australia, ACORN Ltd.

AORN 1997 Maintaining a Sterile Field. Standards, Recommended Practices, and Guidelines. Denver, AORN Inc.

Babbs J Bradley C R 1995 A review of Glutaraldehyde alternatives. British Journal of Theatre Nursing. 5 (7) 20-24

Bennett G 1994 Flash sterilisation, its limitations and recommendations. ACORN Journal. 7 (2) 19-21

Control of Substances Hazardous to Health Regulation 1988

Davis P 1993 Flash sterilisation - the OR experience. ACORN Journal. 6 (1) 27-30

HSE 1997 Glutaraldehyde. CHAN 7. September

Larkin M A 1991 Aseptic technique adherence never goes out of style. AORN Journal. 54 (2) 353-355

Leonard R 1995 BCAM Sterile "a lesson in asepsis". Canadian Operating Room Nursing Journal 13 (3) 23-26

McKay G 1996 To sterilise or disinfect - that is the question. British Journal of Theatre Nursing 5 (12) 13-14

Garner B G 1995 Infection Control. In: Meeker M H & Rothrock J C 1995 Alexander's Care of the Patient in Surgery. (10 Edition) Mosby, St Louis

Menzies D 1995 Glutaraldehyde - controlling the risk to health. British Journal of Theatre Nursing. 4 (11) 13-15

NATN 1988 Aseptic Technique. Principles Of Safe Practice In The Operating Theatre. Harrogate, NATN

NATN 1998 Infection Control. Principles Of Safe Practice In The Perioperative Environment. Harrogate, NATN

NATN 1998 Preparation of Personnel. Principles Of Safe Practice In The Perioperative Environment. Harrogate, NATN

NATN 1998 Scrubbing, Gowning and Gloving.

Principles Of Safe Practice In The Perioperative Environment. Harrogate, NATN

NATN 1998 Trolley Preparation for Surgical Intervention. Principles Of Safe Practice In The Perioperative Environment. Harrogate, NATN

NATN 1998 Use and Handling of Instruments. Principles Of Safe Practice In The Perioperative Environment. Harrogate, NATN

NATN 1998 Visitors to the Perioperative Environment. Principles Of Safe Practice In The Perioperative Environment. Harrogate, NATN

Porteous J Gembey D Dieter M 1996 Bowel technique in the OR. Is it really necessary? Canadian Operating Room Nursing Journal. 14 (1) 11-13

SATS 1997 Back to basic principles, aseptic technique. South African Theatre Sisters Journal. 22 (1) 41-46

Recommendations for Inclusion in Local Policy

The three main areas for consideration when developing local policy are:

    i.   General considerations
    ii.   Equipment safeguards
    iii.   Special considerations

1. General considerations

a. Perioperative staff with infected lesions of the skin or bacterial infections of the upper respiratory system should not participate in any aseptic technique.

b. Staff participating in an aseptic technique should present themselves as recommended in Preparation of Personnel and Scrubbing, Gowning and Gloving, within this section.

c. Personnel participating within sterile procedures must stay within the sterile boundaries, and a wide margin of safety should be given between scrubbed and non scrubbed persons.

d. The environment and all working surfaces must be cleaned in accordance with local infection control policies prior to the commencement of the procedure.

e. All pre-sterilised articles must be checked for damage and expiry date prior to use. Any packs found to be in an unsatisfactory condition must be discarded. Items used within a sterile field must be sterile.

f. Sterile drapes should be used to establish a sterile field.

g. To maintain asepsis it is essential that all staff are aware of the correct method of opening different sterile packages to avoid the contamination of contents.

h. Any dressings must be removed carefully from the wound to prevent scattering of microorganisms into the air. It is recommended that this is carried out by an assistant wearing gloves rather than a scrubbed member of the surgical team. Used and soiled dressings should be discarded immediately and in accordance with local infection control policy.

i. To reduce the risk of airborne cross infection the following should be kept to a minimum: talking, movement, opening and closing doors, exposure of wounds, disturbance of clothing and linen, and number of personnel in the theatre. Care must be taken to maintain the integrity of the sterile field at all times.

j. Every sterile field should be constantly monitored and maintained as sterility cannot be assured without direct observation of the sterile field.

2. Equipment safeguards

The following recommendations are made in order to provide guidelines for the sterilisation and disinfection of supplies and equipment

a. All items should be thoroughly cleaned prior to sterilisation or disinfection, as the reliability of the process is affected by the number, type and inherent resistance of organisms on the item which will be sterilised.

b. The surrounding materials or packaging may interfere with the penetration of a sterilant and therefore all packing should be clean and conform to national guidelines.

c. All articles to be sterilised should be arranged so that all surfaces will be directly exposed to the sterilising agent for the prescribed duration and temperature. To achieve this all instruments should be open and/or unlocked. Instruments must be disassembled where appropriate.

d. Chemical indicators should be used to indicate that items have been effectively exposed to a sterilisation process.

e. The efficiency of the sterilising process should be monitored at regular intervals with reliable biological or thermal indicators.

f. Flash sterilisation should be used for emergency purposes only. Unwrapped instruments and porous items only should be placed in flash sterilisers.

g. Planned preventative maintenance of all sterilisers should be performed according to local policy on a scheduled basis and by a qualified engineer.

3. Special considerations

a. Disinfection is the chemical inactivation of non-sporing organisms. As disinfection is not a means of sterilisation, strict adherence to protocol is necessary for successful disinfection to be achieved.

b. The method of cleaning and the selection of the appropriate chemical disinfectant should take into consideration the physical properties of the item, the manufacturers instructions and the occupational health and safety requirements associated with the disinfectant.

c. The length of time required to achieve disinfection varies, and is dependant on the following factors: the nature of the contaminating microorganisms, the length of exposure to the agent, and the temperature. All disinfectants will cease to be effective after repeated use due to dilution, inactivation and/or instability.

Principles of Safe Practice in The Perioperative Environment

Clinical Practice - *Section 3*

USE AND HANDLING OF INSTRUMENTS

Introduction

Most operating departments use trays of instruments which are prepared, checked and packed by personnel in central supply units.

It is essential that a system is incorporated in the local policy for checking that instruments are decontaminated, in good repair and of an agreed standard, before packing and autoclaving. It is however, possible that some defects may be overlooked, therefore, the scrub person is also responsible for checking surgical instruments prior to the commencement and on the completion of surgical intervention.

The method of cleaning, selection of packing material and method of sterilisation of surgical instruments and other items should be undertaken according to the physical properties of the item and the manufacturer's instruments.

Instruments which are found to be defective must be removed, labelled and sent for repair or replacement in accordance with local policy.

Theatre staff should be aware of the implications of reprocessing surgical instruments as outlined in the Product Liability Act. It is therefore important that all staff involved in instrument processing have full instruction and understanding of the techniques involved.

Theatre staff should be aware of the medico-legal implications of reprocessing items, this including single use items.

BIBLIOGRAPHY

ACORN 1998 Reprocessing of Reusable Items - Cleaning, packing, sterilisation and storage of sterile supplies. Standards, Guidelines and Policy Statements. Australia, ACORN Ltd.

AORN 1997 Care and Cleaning of Surgical Instruments and Powered Equipment. Standards, Recommended Practices and Guidelines. Denver, AORN Inc.

AORN 1997 Selection and Use of Packaging Systems. Standards, Recommended Practices and Guidelines. Denver, AORN Inc.

AORN 1997 Sterilisation in the Practice Setting. Standards, Recommended Practices and Guidelines. Denver, AORN Inc.

Bell S 1998 Multiple Patient Use Versus Single Patient Use Products. British Journal of Theatre Nursing. 8 (1) 1-24

Chadwick S 1994 Event Related Outdating: a fairy tale comes true, Canadian Operating Room Nursing Journal. 12 (4) 22-26

Consumer Protection Act 1987 Part 1: Product Liability

Crow S 1993 Protecting Patients, personnel, instruments in the OR. AORN Journal. 58 (4) 771-774

DesCoteaux J G Poulis E C Julien M Guiduin 1995 Residual organic debris on processed surgical instruments. AORN Journal. 62 (1) 23-30

DOH 1989 A Guide to Good Manufacturing Practice for NHS Sterile Services Departments

Finkelstein L E Mendelson M H Schneider N J 1997 How to safely clean surgical instruments. American Journal of Nursing. 97 (6) 59

Fullbrook S 1998 Medico-legal insights - legal aspects of the re-use of single use items. British Journal of Theatre Nursing. 8 (3) 37-39

ISSM 1984 A Training Handbook for Sterile Supply Staff UK London.

Lamb J Foster S Henderson E Krulicki W 1996 Significant savings achieved by implementing event related outdating. Canadian Operating Room Nursing Journal. 14 (3) 12-14

Malchesky P S Chamberlain V C Scott Connor C Salis B Wallace C 1995 Reprocessing of reusable medical devices. ASAIO Journal. 41 (2) 146-157

MDA Directive 1993 93/42/EEC

MDA Regulations 1994 SI 3017

MDA 1995 The reuse of medical devices supplied for single use only.

DB 9501

MDA 1998 Reporting adverse incidents relating to medical devices.

SN 9801

NATN 1995 Quality Assessment Document (QUAD) Harrogate, NATN

NATN 1997 Universal Precaution and Infection Control in the Perioperative Setting. Harrogate, NATN

NATN 1998 Endoscopes. Infection Control. The Count. Trolley Preparation for Surgical Intervention. Aseptic Technique. Principles Of Safe Practice In The Perioperative Environment. Harrogate, NATN

NATN 1998 Safeguards for Invasive Procedures: The Management of Risks. Harrogate, NATN

Olsen C C 1995 Sutures, Needles, and Instruments. In: Meeker M H and Rothrock J C 1995 Alexander's Care of the Patient in Surgery. (10th Edition) Mosby, St Louis

Raltz S L Kozarek R A Pethigal P A Moorhouse M A Merrian L D 1995 Reusable biopsy forceps : a cost effective measure for the endoscopy suite. Gastroenterology Nursing. 18 (5) 167-70

Sales of Goods Act 1979

Science Journal 1995 Lubricants and HIV Science 26 9 (5 229) 1343

Smith C D 1994 Event-related sterility - clinical issues. AORN Journal. 59 (6) 1313-1314

Supply of Goods and Services Act 1998

Taylor M Campbell C Surgical Preparation In: Clarke P Jones J (Eds) 1998 Brigden's Operating Department Practice. Edinburgh, Churchill Livingstone

The Case Against Re-use, The Medical and Surgical Products Liaison Group.

Recommendations for Inclusion in Local Policy

The three main areas for consideration are:

1. Care of Instruments
2. General Safeguards
3. Storage of Instruments

1. Care of Instruments

a. Staff involved in the cleaning and packing process of instruments must undertake to use universal blood and body substance isolation precautions.

b. In order to prevent damage, instruments must only be used for the purpose for which they are designed. (e.g. osteotomes are not levers) Proper selection requires a general understanding of surgical procedures and a knowledge of anatomy.

c. In order to prevent corrosion or damage, instruments must not be immersed in:

i. Saline.
ii. Hypochlorite.
iii. Chemical disinfectants.

d. To prevent damage, delicate instruments should be handled with care and separated from other instruments.

e. Specialised instruments should be regularly checked by an appropriately trained person. Specialist equipment should be made available to check the integrity of diathermy cables and instruments.

2. General Safeguards

a. Regular inspection of all instruments should be made by an appropriately qualified person.

b. In order to maintain asepsis, instruments found to be contaminated with dried blood or body tissue prior to surgery must be discarded. If found on a tray of instruments, the whole tray must be discarded and the incident reported to the appropriate person.

c. If, on opening a tray of instruments, any areas are damp or drops of moisture are observed, the whole tray must be discarded and the incident reported.

d. Each tray of instruments should contain an instrument check list, which incorporates the information necessary for a recorded programme of use.

e. Instruments must be accounted for at all times during a surgical procedure.

f. The scrub person should ensure that instruments are handled in such a manner as to avoid personal injury, injury to the patient or to other members of the surgical team.

g. Special care should be taken with sharp instruments (e.g. scalpels and loaded needle holders). It is strongly recommended that all sharp instruments are transferred between staff in a receiver.

h. Instruments must not be allowed to rest directly on the patient, which could cause:

i. Injury to the patient.

ii. Damages to the drapes. Consideration should be given to the use of appropriate additional sterile surfaces (e.g. Mayo tables, magnetic pads).

i. Instruments which have been taken directly from an autoclave into the operating theatre or lay-up room must be allowed to cool naturally before use.

j. Organisations and individuals which are party to the reprocessing of items owe the patient a duty of care to do no harm, which means ensuring that each and every item is sterile, safe and fit for its purpose. The person who undertakes the sterilisation is accountable. This applies whether the item is a single or multi use item.

k. Items sterilised on site should be labelled with load control identification to allow items to be retrieved in the event of sterilisation malfunction or failure. Accurate records must be kept. Record of products used should also be recorded in a patient's notes to ensure that all items used on a patient can be traced from beginning to finish.

3. Storage of instruments

a. The storage area should be clean, dry and free of dust.

b. All storage surfaces should be smooth, non-porous and capable of being easily cleaned.

c. Sterile items should be protected from direct sunlight.

d. The temperature of the storage area should range between 22 C and 24 C with a relative humidity of 35% - 68%.

e. Perioperative personnel should have the knowledge and skills related to the handling of sterile items.

f. Sterilised items should be transferred to and from storage areas on clean, specifically designated trolleys.

g. All sterile items should have an event related shelf life. The length of time an item can be considered sterile is referred to as the shelf life. The event related outdating theory is based on the assumption that if items are properly cleaned, wrapped, sterilised, stored and handled they can remain sterile indefinitely unless the integrity of the packaging is compromised. Therefore, the shelf life of an item is dependent on storage, handling and type of packaging material.

Principles of Safe Practice in The Perioperative Environment

Clinical Practice - *Section 3*

UNIVERSAL PRECAUTIONS

Introduction

The risk of exposure to blood and body fluids is recognised as being very high for those working in the perioperative setting.

In today's world, the system of selective or diagnosis driven infection control policies are no longer appropriate. Within care settings there is no quick way of identifying sero-positive HIV, HBV and/or HCV patients, therefore treating all patients as potentially infected is a sensible informed professional approach.

The philosophy of universal precautions (or "standard" precautions) recognises that it is the **task** or **activity** that is to be completed that should be assessed and **not** the individual who is to receive the care.

As all patients have the right to be treated with dignity and respect, the use of universal precautions eliminates the risk of random inappropriate practice and permits the staff to deliver high standards of safe care. By practising in such a way, staff protect their patients, themselves and other members of the caring team.

BIBLIOGRAPHY

ACORN 1998 Standard and Additional Precautions in the Operating Suite. Standards, Guidelines and Policy Statement. Australia, ACORN Ltd

Advisory Committee on Dangerous Pathogens, 1995 Protection against blood-borne infections in the workplace - HIV and Hepatitis, HMSO

Aids Reference Manual 1996 NAM Publications (19th Edition) London

AORN, 1997 Environmental cleaning in the surgical practice setting. Standards, Recommended Practices and Guidelines. Denver, AORN Inc.

AORN 1997 Universal precautions in the perioperative setting. Standards Recommended Practices and Guidelines. Denver, AORN Inc.

Bell S 1998 Multiple patient use versus single patient use products. British Journal of Theatre Nursing. 8 (1) 1 - 24

Borton D 1997 Isolation Precautions. Nursing. 27 (1) 49-51

Dyke M 1996 Why not wear gloves. British Journal of Theatre Nursing. 6 (6) 14-17

Environmental Protection Act 1990

Fish J 1992 An alternative to swab racks. Nursing Standard. 7 (3) 55-56

Fogg D M 1997 OR Expansions reuse of single use medical devices: universal standard and transmission based precautions. AORN Journal. 65 (3) 636-639

Health and Safety at Work Act 1974

Howard-Philpott J Casewell M 1994 Hospital Infection Control Policies and Practical Procedures. London, WB Saynders Co Ltd

ICNA 1997 Guidelines for Hand Hygiene. Derbyshire, Deb Ltd.

Lamb A 1992 The swab rack - an outdated ritual British Journal of Theatre Nursing. 2 (2) 14-17

Mumford M 1991 Swab racks are an old fashioned idea. British Journal of Theatre Nursing. 1 (9) 20-21

NATN 1992 Universal precautions for the handling of blood and body fluids. Principles Of Safe Practice In The Operating Theatre. Harrogate, NATN

NATN 1997 Universal Precautions and Infection

Control in the Perioperative Setting. Harrogate, NATN

NATN 1998 Infection Control. Principles Of Safe Practice In The Perioperative Environment. Harrogate, NATN

NATN 1998 Safeguards for Invasive Procedures : The Management of Risks. Harrogate, NATN

NHS Estates 1994 A Strategic Guide to Clinical Waste Management

Norman A 1995 A comparison of face masks and visors for the scrub team. British Journal of Theatre Nursing. 5 (2) 10-13

Ronk L L Girard N J 1994 Risk Perception Universal Precautions Compliance. AORN Journal. 59 (1) 253-266

RCN 1992 Introduction to Methicillin-resistant Staphylococcus Aureus. London, RCN

RCN 1995 Infection Control in Hospitals. London, RCN

RCN 1997 Universal Precautions. London, RCN

Taylor M 1993 Universal precautions in the Operating Department. British Journal of Theatre Nursing. 2 (10) 4-7

DOH 1990 Guidance for Clinical Health Care Workers: Protection against Infection with HIV and Hepatitis Viruses. London, HMSO

Wicker C P 1991 Universal Precautions: Infection Control in a High Risk Environment. British Journal of Theatre Nursing. 1 (9) 16-18

Williams M 1996 Infection control and universal precautions. British Journal of Theatre Nursing. 6 (2) 8-9

Recommendations for Inclusion in Local Policy

The practitioner must assess **risk factors** inherent in each procedure. The type of protective clothing that is worn and the precautions that are taken are dependent on the risk of contamination with blood and body fluids associated with specific procedures.

1. Management Considerations

The overall function of an infection control policy is to help minimise the risk of infection transmission to either patient or staff.

a. Infection control is an issue of health and safety. It comes within the remit of the Health and Safety at Work Act 1974, and is still the essential reference point when considering health and safety at work. The basic objective is to ensure staff are protected while at work.

b. Managers must ensure that all staff are familiar with the precautions laid down in local infection control policies. Any changes that may be made to comply with legislation or recommendations must be made known to staff and implemented.

c. An occupational health programme of Hepatitis B vaccination is essential and must be available to all staff who work within the perioperative environment.

d. Any concerns which staff may have with occupational exposure to blood-borne pathogens should be addressed to the occupational health department or another medical source in accordance with local policy.

e. Perioperative environment environmental standards must comply with the DOH guidelines, and it is the responsibility of all theatre personnel to ensure that these standards are monitored and maintained. Appropriate documentation should be completed.

2. Universal Precautions

Perioperative personnel must assess the risk factors involved in each procedure. Many of the following points should be practised for all patients:

a. Effective communication within the clinical area must always be practised to ensure a thorough knowledge of the patient and their condition.

b. The patient must be provided with clean bed/trolley linen and theatre gown just before going to theatre.

c. The patient should be greeted and provided with respect and consideration through their perioperative phase.

d. In specific cases staff should use appropriate respirators which filter inspired air.

e. A minimum number of personnel should be maintained within the operating room.

f. There should be a restriction on personnel movement and talking.

g. The doors to the operating room should be keep shut whenever possible.

h. An effective air-changing/ventilation system should be used and maintained.

i. Soiled linen and waste must be disposed of carefully and in accordance with Health and Safety Commission guidelines.

j. If disposable anaesthetic breathing circuits are not used then the circuit should be changed and cleaned according to local policy and any filters used, renewed.

k. All other re-usable equipment should be decontaminated according to local policy

Specific universal precautions that are recommended for local implementation are:

(1) Skin

i. All cuts or skin abrasions should be covered with quality waterproof dressings.

ii. Contact with blood/body fluids must be avoided if compromised by a hand or arm skin disorder.

(2) Hand Washing

i. Effective hand washing techniques must always be used.

ii. The use of gloves does not preclude the need for hand washing before and after patient contact.

(3) Gloves

i. High quality gloves should always be worn when contact with a patient's blood/body fluids is anticipated.

(4) Eyes and Mouth

i. The risk of splash or aerosol must always be assessed and either mask and goggles or full face visors worn.

ii. Hand to mouth contact should be avoided.

(5) Gowns

i. Whenever contact with blood/body fluids is anticipated water repellent clothing should be worn.

ii. Circulating staff should wear gloves, plastic aprons and eye protection whenever there is an assessed risk of possible contamination.

iii. Additional measures may be deemed necessary if there is a risk of excessive blood/body fluid loss, e.g. cover operating table with non permeable sheet, use fluid collecting drapes, use floor suction apparatus.

(6) Sharps

i.   Adherence to local policy is necessary for the correct use and disposal of sharps. This will include the following:

   a) Use of an appropriate instrument for careful application and removal of a surgical blades to and from a handle.

   b) Provision of a 'neutral zone' where sharps can be placed in a receiver for safe use and retrieval during procedures.

   c) Careful, correct disposal of sharps at the end of procedure.

   d) Needles should never be re-sheathed unless an appropriate device is used to facilitate this.

(7) Spillage

i.   There must be a local policy on dealing with spillages within the perioperative environment.

(8) Swabs

i.   Whatever local policy is in use for count procedures, practitioners must ensure that swabs are safely contained, whilst easily accounted for.

(9) Sharps Injury/Conjunctiva/mucous membrane splash

In the event of an injury the following actions should be immediately taken:

i.   Encourage bleeding if the skin has been punctured.

ii.   Wash the area with running water and soap.

iii. Wash eye splash with tap water or saline.

iv.   If accidental inoculation of blood from a patient known or suspected to be HCV positive occurs, a blood sample from the patient should be stored.

v.   Report to the occupational health department or other medical source immediately, as per local policy.

vi.   Advise line manager of incident and document nature of event.

(10) Waste Disposal

i.   All clinical refuse must be placed in appropriate sacks, as per local policy, and sealed prior to incineration.

ii.   All used linen must be placed in bags, designated for this purpose as per local policy, sealed and placed in appropriate laundry sacks prior to dispatch. Used instruments should be dispatched to the appropriate processing area according to local policy.

Principles of Safe Practice in
The Perioperative Environment
Clinical Practice - *Section 3*

PROCEDURES RELATED TO ORGAN DONATION

Introduction

During the last two decades, transplantation has developed rapidly in the UK. Multi-organ donation has become commonplace and is widely accepted by professionals and the public alike. Heart, lung, liver and kidney transplants now have an excellent one and five year survival rate. Pancreatic and small bowel transplantation are also fast developing.

The potential organ donor is a patient in whom brain stem death has been confirmed, but still has a beating heart and who is maintained on artificial ventilation.

There has been widespread acceptance of the guidelines for brain death and for the criteria that allows the patient to become a candidate as a beating heart cadaver donor since the 1970's.

A code of practice was issued by the DOH in December 1979, and was designed to allay public fears about the circumstances in which organs may be removed from dead patients for the purpose of transplantation. The two principles of the code are to:

a. set out the precise procedure which should be followed by doctors in deciding whether a person is clinically dead,

b. set out the manner in which doctors should properly approach relatives for permission to remove organs.

A code of criteria for the diagnosis of brain death was drawn up by the Royal Colleges in 1976. Their code for transplants, issued in 1978, built on the previous criteria, is intended to reassure public fears about the time of death. The time of death should be recorded as the time when death was conclusively established and **not** when ventilation was withdrawn or the heart beat ceased.

Organ transplants are regulated by the Human Tissue Act of 1961. This act provides for the use of the bodies of deceased persons for therapeutic and medical examination and research purposes.

The Human Organ Transplants Act of 1989 places restrictions upon transplants between live persons. It can impose certain criminal offences and was drafted to address problems posed by trade in organs. This Act does not apply to blood or bone marrow transplantation.

Prior to the removal of any organ, the following is required to have been established by the regional donor transplant co-ordinator:

a. Diagnosis of brain stem death.

b. Confirmation of a lack of objection to organ donation from the nearest relative.

c. Screening for Hepatitis B and C, HIV, cytomegalovirus and history of malignancy.

d. Notification to the coroner if necessary.

Matching criteria should include:

a. Compatible blood group.

b. Height and weight.

c. Comparable cytomegalovirus antibody status (lung transplantation).

Donor organ procurement can be an emotive subject for perioperative staff and it is therefore essential that operating departments have a clearly defined policy with outlines of procedures, to help avoid confusion and anxiety.

BIBLIOGRAPHY

Callender S Mathews S 1998 Caring for the carers during transplant surgery. British Journal of Theatre Nursing. 8 (1) 5-12

Crombie A Nicolls J 1992 Organ donation and the theatre nurse. British Journal of Theatre Nursing. 2 (2) 4-6

DOH 1979 A Code of Practice including the Diagnosis of Brain Death Cadaveric Organs for Transplantation. London

Directory of Operating Theatres & Departments of Surgery 1998 United Kingdom Transplant Support Service Authority. 1-26. Cambridge, CMA Medical Data

Dimond B 1990 Legal Aspects of Nursing. Lancaster, Quay Publishing Ltd.

Finch J 1994 Organ transplants and disposal of the human body. Spellers Law Relating to Hospital (7th Edition), Chapman and Hall Medical

Human Organ Transplantation Act 1989

Human Tissue Act 1961

Ledbetter A K 1995 Trauma Surgery. In: Meeker R H and Rothrock J C 1995 Alexander's Care of the Patient. (10th Edition) Mosby, St Louis

Lloyd-Jones H 1992 A cardiac programme - the nurses role. British Journal of Theatre Nursing. 2 (4) 21-23

Lloyd-Jones H Wheeldon D R Smith J A Potter C D Wallwork J Large S R 1996 An Approach to the Retrieval of Thoracic Organs for Transplantation. AORN Journal. 63 (2) 416-426

NATN, 1992 Procedures related to organ donation. Principles Of Safe Practice In The Operating Theatre. Harrogate, NATN

Page S 1996 Responses of perioperative nurses to organ procurement surgery. Canadian Operating Room Nursing Journal. 14 (4) 9-11

Stewart R 1994 Transplantation issues in the United Kingdom. Intensive and Critical Care Nursing. 10 (2) 105-106

Sque M Payne S 1994 Gift exchange theory: a critique in relation to organ transplantation. Journal of Advanced Nursing. 19 (1) 45-51

United Kingdom Transplant Co-ordinators Association 1994 Standards of Practice for Procurement Co-ordinators. Birmingham, UKTCA

United Kingdom Transplant Support Service Authority 1997 User's bulletin No 23. Spring

Watson D S 1995 Contemporary Issues. In: Meeker R H and Rothrock J C 1995 Alexander's Care of the Patient. (10th Edition) Mosby, St Louis

Whyte A 1997 The Ultimate Gift. Nursing Times. 93 (27) 26-29

Recommendations for Inclusion in Local Policy

1. Organ Procurement Procedures

a. As transplantation techniques have improved, there has been an increase in the number of organs that are able to be retrieved from each donor and this in turn, has made the organisation of organ donation procedures more complex. The transplant co-ordinator is therefore a key figure in the organisation of organ donation. They liaise between the donor theatre team, transplants teams and the intensive care unit staff, striving to minimise difficulties so that the procedure can be viewed as a positive experience for relatives and all personnel involved.

b. The timing of the organ procurement procedures are usually calculated to co-ordinate with the recipient procedures. The transplant team will require medical details about the donor, and the transplant co-ordinator will be able to provide guidance about the information normally requested for each type of transplant.

c. Although the transplant procurement teams are largely self sufficient and bring with them the instruments, drugs and perfusion fluids necessary for their procedure, the donor theatre will need to provide certain items and equipment. This may include, but is not limited to:

    i. Trolleys, bowls stands.

    ii. Basic general instruments.

    iii. Gowns, drapes, swabs, sutures.

    iv. Suction, diathermy.

    v. Large quantities of crushed ice.

    vi. Perioperative personnel.

d. The United Kingdom Transplant Support Service Authority (UKTSSA) is a special health authority of the NHS and it provides a service to the organ transplant units in the UK and the Republic of Ireland and is responsible for maintaining records of all patients who are waiting for organ transplantation. It provides a 24 hour support service for matching and allocating donor organs, and is also a focal point for information on transplant matters and is available as an enquiry service.

2. Useful Addresses

The Information Executive
UK Transplant Support Service Authority
Fox Den Road
Stoke Gifford
Bristol BS34 8RR

UK Transplant Co-ordinators Association
UKTCA Secretariat
PO 6300
Birmingham B15 2RN

3. Considerations for the Transplant Team

a. All procedures during procurement surgery must adhere to the local hospital policies and must meet nationally recognised standards.

b. It is important that all procedures are afforded the same professionalism as other surgical procedures.

c. Effective communication and feedback to the donor unit is important so that perioperative staff can identify with the more positive aspects of transplantation surgery and to prevent the feeling of isolation.

4. Tissue Donation

a. Occasionally other tissues are donated. These include heart values, bone samples and skin; the transplant co-ordinator will advise on the process of retrieval. Samples of tissue for research may also be taken with the relatives permission, and this consent will need to be clearly recorded in the notes.

b. Samples of lymph node and spleen are taken at the time of kidney retrieval and are used for tissue typing. Permission will need to be sought for this routine procedure.

5. Last Offices

a. Once the retrieval teams have finished and the surgeons have closed the abdomen and chest appropriately, last offices can be performed according to local policy. Wherever possible, the personal wishes of the donor or their relatives should be respected.

b. If a post mortem is required, this will be arranged with the pathologist. The relatives should be reassured that organ donation will not delay any funeral arrangements, and should be encouraged to view the body post donation if they wish. However, they should be made aware if there is to be an inquest or post mortem as this may delay the funeral.

6. Other considerations for the Donor Procurement Units

a. It is helpful to identify a member of staff who will meet the procurement team/s on arrival and introduce them to the environment, thus streamlining arrival and departure.

b. Organ procurement surgery can be an emotive procedure, and perioperative nurses who participate in the procurement phase of organ donation can be subjected to stressful emotions. Consideration must therefore be given to the provision of support programmes. Counselling support, stress management and education of staff regarding the concept of brain stem death and the purpose of the operative procedures will help the perioperative staff to deliver an effective service.

Principles of Safe Practice in The Perioperative Environment

Staff Welfare and Development - *Section 4*

Reviewers

Craig Bibby RGN FETC
Theatre Education Manager
Plymouth Hospital NHS Trust

Martin Hind RGN DPSN Bsc(Hons) PGDE MSc
Senior Lecturer in Critical Care
Bournemouth University

Lesley Fudge BA(Hons) RGN ONC Dip Eur Hum(Open)
Theatre Manager
Frenchay Hospital

Principles of Safe Practice in
The Perioperative Environment
Staff Development and Welfare - *Section 4*

GOOD EMPLOYMENT PRACTICE (PERSONNEL GUIDELINES)

Introduction

This principle outlines a concise overview of current employment legislation in order that all perioperative staff understand their employment entitlements and what their employers can expect of them.

The aim of all organisations including health care providers may be described as the achievement of identified aims and objectives by using available resources as effectively as possible. People are often considered to be the most important and valuable resource within the Health Service despite being the least predictable. It then follows that effective management of people must be fundamental in achieving the objectives of the organisation.

In most organisations such as the NHS or other health care providers this is usually undertaken by the 'line manager' with contributions or advice from the Directorate of Human Resources (personnel), working within both national and european employment legislation and local policies and guidelines.

Local policies generally outline current legislation, local agreements and management guidelines that have been implemented to govern the conduct of employers in relation to employees. Such documents should be freely available to staff and should be regularly updated as changes in conditions of service occur.

BIBLIOGRAPHY

Atherton S 1996 The effectiveness of Personnel Management in the NHS.

Beardwell I Holden L 1994 Human resource Management: A Contemporary Perspective. Pitman

Cumming M W 1986 The Theory and Practice of Personnel Management. W Heinnemann Ltd.

Dimond B 1995 Contracts of Emploment, the law and the nurse. British Journal of Nursing. 4 (12) 674-675

DOH 1992 Management of Health and Safety at Work Act Regulations. SI 2051 London, HMSO

Employment Protection Act 1975

Health and Safety at Work Act 1974

Hodgson J 1993 Employment Law for Nurses. Lancaster, Quay Publishing Ltd.

Lewis D 1990 Essentials of Employment Law. Institute of Personnel Management

NATN 1990 Operating Department: Identifying Non-Medical Skill Mix. Harrogate, NATN

Rehabilitation of Offenders Act 1974

Sex Discrimination Act 1975

Trade Union and Labour Relation Act 1974

Waud C 1992 Employment Law. London, Michael O' Mara Books Ltd.

Recommendations for Inclusion in Local Policy

Good employment practice will encompass and provide protocols and standards for the following:

1. Workforce planning and job analysis
2. Job analysis and evaluation
3. Employment legislation
4. Recruitment and selection procedures
5. Conditions of service (contracts)
6. Training and education
7. Disciplinary and grievance procedures
8. Counselling and welfare

1. Workforce planning and job analysis

In practice workforce planning is concerned with the demand and supply of labour by examining workloads and estimating staffing levels. This includes identifying skills required to undertake a task in a safe and competent manner. Workforce planning is a continuous process and should have a clearly identified monitoring process. Any organisational system has to be based on analyses of demand and supply and the plans and decisions which follow these analyses.

2. Job analysis and evaluation

Linked and integrated into workforce planning is the need to conduct job analysis and evaluation throughout the organisation.

This is a key function of management and is essential for all processes leading to the effective performance of work. It is also a pre-requisite for job evaluation, and for establishing roles and relationships within the workplace. It is essential that all managers both understand and skilfully apply principles to practice. In conducting this exercise the following should be examined.

    a.   Job description
    b.   Job specification
    c.   Person specification

a. Job description

This is a statement of component tasks, duties, objectives, standards and environmental circumstances of a job.

b. Job specification

This specifies the skills, knowledge and attitudes required to perform a job.

c. Person specification

This is an interpretation of the job specification in terms of the kind of person needed to perform a job effectively. Its main use is in personnel selection.

3. Employment legislation

This is very complex, it is constantly changing and therefore should be adjusted accordingly. This section should be divided into the following headings:

a. Trade Union and Labour Relations Act 1974.

This must include information and guidelines on purpose, right to union membership, closed shops, unfair dismissal, record of dismissal and collective agreements.

b. The Employment Protection Act 1975

This represents the second stage of the Government's programme and aims to:

i. Strengthen collective bargaining.

ii. Improve security and rights of employees.

iii. Promote the concept of independent trade unions.

Local policy must include information on Advisory Conciliation and Arbitration Services (ACAS), Guarantee Payments 1977, eligibility, medical suspension, maternity pay, contracts of employment and redundancies.

c. Rehabilitation of Offenders Act 1974

This aims to:

i. Rehabilitate offenders who have not been re-convicted for a certain period of time.

ii. Punish certain unauthorised disclosures of an individual's previous convictions.

iii. Extend the rules regarding defamation.

Local policy must include information on:

Aims, definitions of excluded convictions, rehabilitation periods and the NHS position on employment.

d. Health and Safety Act 1974

The Act aims to provide the legislative framework to promote, stimulate and encourage high standards of health and safety at work. The employer should have a clearly defined health and safety policy that clearly outlines information and procedure on the law, manufacturers and suppliers position, enforcement of the Act and manufacturers and suppliers reporting and first aid facilities.

e. The Sex Discrimination Act 1975

The Act makes sex discrimination unlawful in employment, training and education and includes information on provisions of the Act. Discrimination in employment, exceptions to the Act, midwifery, advertising, reverse discrimination and actions that should be taken in the event of non-compliance must all be included in the employer's policy.

f. Equal opportunities

A statement of intent for the organisation should be clearly stated with a code of practice on recruitment and selection, employment and training and monitoring of the processes designed to identify non-compliance.

4. Recruitment and selection of staff

How an organisation presents itself in terms of public image can determine the quality of staff it is able to recruit. It is critical in providing suitable applicants to fill posts. Recruitment and selection must be an efficient systematic process, which enables the optimum choice, otherwise the whole process will have been neither cost effective nor efficient in terms of resources.

The process should include:

a. The extent of vacancies following a job analysis.

b. The potential source of labour.

c. The preparation and publication of information including an explicit job description, personnel specification, appropriate application form, and information (marketing) about the employing organisation.

d. The process and assessment of applications; to include the short-listing procedures, interview format and dates. Processing of references and occupational health screening.

e. The application process including interview format and results (time scale).

5. Conditions of service

It is important for each employee to understand their exact conditions of service and this should be identified within a contract of employment or letter of appointment. The contract should include details about salary, leave entitlement, sickness policy, period of notice for termination of employment and disciplinary and grievance procedures.

6. Training and education

Employers depend on the quality of their employee's ability to achieve organisational goals and targets. Employees, also have developmental needs and individual goals. In order to meet these, there needs to be a process where the achievement of goals can be measured and recorded. Individual performance review and clinical supervision can be used to meet the needs of the employer and the employee.

a. Induction programme for all new staff

    All new members of staff require a period of support for induction and orientation when starting a new post. This should include induction to the organisation and the working environment. The new employee should have a point of contact during this period. This should be an experienced practitioner who acts as a mentor or facilitator.

b. Staff development system

    All perioperative environments must have a comprehensive 'in-house' multi-professional training programme. The organisation should have policies that ensure each individual is prepared and channelled into the most effective area of service. Flexible positive measures must be available to enable a person to reach their full potential within the organisation. A system of individual performance review is integral to this need.

7. Disciplinary and grievance procedures

Just as we must recognise effort, so the organisation is required to ensure that line managers know how to pursue redress for a grievance and how the disciplinary machinery functions within the organisation. This should also incorporate the process and time frame for moving from the initial to the final stage and the employees' rights of appeal and for representation within this framework.

8. Counselling and welfare

There are times within any organisation when people need help either with their personal life or with career development. It is the responsibility of every manager to undertake this role as and when necessary. In some instances it may not be appropriate for managers to undertake this role because of the confidential nature and sensitivity of individuals needs. Therefore it is an essential part of every organisation to have professional counsellors available to assist with personal and professional issues which will effect job performance e.g. occupational health. This is particularly true in the highly stressed and technical environment of perioperative care.

Principles of Safe Practice in The Perioperative Environment

Staff Development and Welfare - *Section 4*

EDUCATION AND TRAINING

Introduction

The provision of a measurable standard of preoperative care that meets identified quality targets can only be achieved if staff who deliver that care, have acquired and developed the necessary skills and competence to perform the role for which they were employed.

Ideally, all qualified staff employed within the perioperative environment would hold a nationally recognised qualification.

> The English, Scottish, Welsh and Northern Irish National Boards all offer courses that lead to qualifications in perioperative care.
> An extensive list is available from the relevant Board.

> An NVQ level 2 in Operating Department Practice may be accessed by nursing auxiliaries and health care assistants.

In reality there is insufficient access to relevant courses to meet the demands of employers. Consequently many nursing staff are employed and continue to be educated 'in-house' to fulfil the needs of the service.

The introduction of the Higher Award under the Framework for continuing Education (UKCC 1991) has led to these courses being offered at diploma and degree level as a foundation for advanced practice. Some universities have an entry requirement that demands previous experience prior to accessing these courses.

Insufficient numbers of Operating Department Practitioners are being employed to meet the demands of the service and consequently many nursing staff are employed and trained 'in-house' to fulfil this demand.

The NVQ Level 3 in Operating Department Practice (ODP) has led to the need for the development of experienced perioperative staff in the assessment for competence to the National Standards. Resources must be available to allow staff to acquire the Training and Development Lead Body (TDLB) Awards D32/33 and to participate in assessments.

Regular audit of clinical practice areas that accommodate learners is integral to the quality of the learning experiences offered. NVQ, ODP courses are internally and externally verified. Perioperative departments should collaborate with education providers to ensure this happens on a regular basis.

BIBLIOGRAPHY

AAGBI 1998 Assistance for the Anaesthetist. London, The Association of Anaesthetists of Great Britain and Northern Ireland

Benner P 1984 From Novice to Expert, London. Addison Wesley

ENB 1990 A New Structure for Professional Development. London, English National Board

Control of Substances Hazards to Health Regulations 1988

DOH 1989 Working for Patients, Education and Training. Working Paper 10. London, HMSO

NATN 1995 Supporting Learner Nurses in the Operating Department. Harrogate, NATN

NATN 1996 Developing the role of the Support Worker in the Operating Department. Harrogate, NATN

NATN 1998 Professional Development and You. Harrogate, NATN

Nicklin and Kenworthy 1996 Teaching and Assessing in Nursing Practice. An experimental Approach. London, Baillierre-Tindall

Quinn F 1995 The Principles and Practice of Nurse Education. (3rd Edition) London, Chapman and Hall

Schon D A 1982 The Reflective Practitioner. How Professionals Think in Action. New York, Arena Basic Books

UKCC 1986 Project 2000 A New Preparation for Practice. London, UKCC

UKCC 1992 Code of Professional Conduct. (3rd edition) London, UKCC

UKCC 1992 The Scope of Professional Practice. London, UKCC

UKCC 1994 The Future for Professional Practice. The Councils Standards for Education and Practice. London, UKCC

UKCC 1997 PREP and You. London, UKCC

Recommendations for Inclusion in Local Policy

There are 6 main areas for consideration and these are:

1. Educational support
2. Orientation and induction
3. Resources
4. Assessment
5. Professional development
6. Pre-registration learners

1. Educational support

a. It is essential that there is active educational support within all areas of perioperative care as these are recognised as specialist areas of care.

It must be remembered that in order for this strategy to succeed it is imperative that there is firm commitment to education and training from management at all levels.

b. The resources required to fulfil the educational support for learners of all grades will depend on:

   i. The size of the department

   ii. The number of staff and other learners within the clinical areas

   iii. Staff and other learners individual educational needs

c. It is strongly recommended that the identified education co-ordinator should contribute, participate and advise on all aspects of clinical practice and organisational issues.

d. It is essential that there are close links with providers of health care education including universities, institutes of health studies, local colleges, providers of ODP and health care NVQs and providers of in-house education such as management or information technology training.

e. The provision of support for all staff and other learners (e.g. pre registration students) is essential in the clinical environment to enable the effective ongoing development and education of all staff to take place.

f. Encouragement to join a professional body such as NATN and participate in local and national activities.

2. Orientation

a. It is essential that every operating department develops an orientation programme for all new staff, regardless of their role or grade, that can be adapted to meet their individual needs.

   i. This orientation programme should be based on the individuals job profile and appraisal.

   ii. It should include statutory information on procedures in case of fire, health considerations (including manual handling and COSHH) and the availability of occupational health support. Many employers provide a generic induction programme for all new employees covering some or all of these issues.

b. Each new member of staff, of whatever grade, should be allocated to a preceptor or mentor, who will offer support and monitor performance during the induction or educational period. The provision of a clinical supervisor in line with UKCC guidelines is necessary to ensure development and that the employee can meet laid out performance standards.

c. Support for new members of staff should be sufficient to ensure that patient care is not compromised. Resources should be such that individuals are not placed in a position that causes them to question their ability to:

   i. Deliver care of an appropriate standard because of a lack of knowledge or competence

   ii. Feel isolated or unsupported and that their professional accountability is compromised.

d. The induction should include information relating to the organisation. Departmental protocols and procedures should be accessible within the department and outlined within the induction package.

e. Periodic review and development of the orientation programme is essential to ensure maximum benefit to new staff and the organisation.

f. The development of relevant documentation to record and monitor processes is essential.

3. Resources

a. There should be a quiet area set aside for books, journals, videos etc. for personal study, tutorials etc.

b. Staff should be encouraged to use this area and other on-site resources whenever possible and to contribute new information, articles, research reports etc.

c. A specific budget should be identified to ensure that specialist reference text is provided for staff use in each area or care.

4. Assessment

a. It should not be assumed that experienced perioperative staff have the necessary skills or knowledge required when transferring to a new area of care (e.g. orthopaedics to ophthalmics). Careful assessment of basic skills and a period of orientation are essential before competence can be achieved.

b. Experienced theatre staff should be encouraged to undertake relevant and recognised courses on teaching and assessing in the clinical areas that will meet the needs of all learners in that area.

c. It is essential that assessors and candidates are aware of the implications of an individual assessment before it is undertaken. Reference should be made to the assessment systems of individual courses.

5. Professional development

a. Resources should be available for professional development of all staff working in the perioperative environment.

b. Trained staff should be encouraged to participate in continuing professional development programmes and management courses. Development needs should be identified through individual performance review.

c. Support for individual nurses in meeting the Post Registration Education for Practice (PREP) requirements should be available, allowing them to identify their needs and record their personal and professional development.

d. The participation of experienced staff in education and training programmes and the development of protocols and procedures should be encouraged.

e. The introduction of new equipment and techniques requires training and information to be given to staff. Suppliers involved are obliged to provide training and this should be arranged for all staff who will participate in it's use.

6. Pre-registration learners

a. The term pre-registration learners is used to describe students of nursing and student ODPs.

b. All basic learners should be granted supernumerary status and allocated to an identified trained staff member who will act as the clinical assessor and mentor.

c. In order that pre-registration students may develop a greater understanding of the total care provision afforded to the surgical patient, it is essential that they undertake a perioperative allocation within the programme. Therefore, it is essential that representation is made to the course providers at a local level to encourage Dip HE nursing students to undertake these placements.

d. Operating department nursing is highly specialised and can prove to be stressful to pre-registration students therefore:

    i. It is essential that a pre-placement orientation programme is devised which includes patient and staff safety, control of infection and patient confidentiality and advocacy, within all areas of care and that clear aims and objectives are presented, in order that the learners are able to make the best use of their placement.

    ii. The experience should be pro-active and not observational and the learners should be encouraged to practice basic perioperative skills and care under the guidance of their assessor or mentor.

    iii Comprehensive evaluation for the placement is essential to ensure that maximum benefit for the learners and a dynamic approach of evaluation will ensure the developments of the placement content.

Principles of Safe Practice in The Perioperative Environment

Staff Development and Welfare - *Section 4*

POTENTIAL HAZARDS TO STAFF

Introduction

This principle begins with the clarification of functions and roles in order that the local protocols and procedures may be developed, this ensuring that staff of all grades understand clearly their individual responsibilities related to health and safety issues.

In addition, it should be noted that loss of Crown Immunity has had a considerable effect in this area.

Two corporate bodies have been established in accordance with the Health and Safety at Work Act 1974. These are the Health and Safety Commission (HSC) and the Health and Safety Executive (HSE).

General Functions

1. To assist and encourage persons to comply with the general purposes of the Act.

2. To make appropriate arrangements for the conduct of research providing training and information in connection with those purposes and to encourage research, training and the provision of information by others.

3. To make arrangements for ensuring that government departments, employers, employees, trade unions, employers' organisations and others concerned with health and safety at work, are provided with an information and advisory service and are kept informed and adequately advised on such matters.

4. To submit proposals for making of regulations. (extract from Croner's 1989).

Employer

The employer's duty is to provide and maintain systems of work that are as far as reasonably practicable, safe and without risks to health. The employer needs to liaise closely with all other departments as there is a responsibility to other disciplines using the department.

The employer must ensure that all policies relating to health and safety are easily accessible at all times to all members of the staff.

Employee

The employee's duty is to abide by those systems and to implement their recommendations in order to protect him or herself and his or her work colleagues and clients.

In addition employees must advise their employer of new developments, updates and recommendations of specific dangers that relate to safe practice within the working environment.

Hazard

A hazard represents the existence of an unsafe system of work, which encompasses a risk to the health and safety of an employee, patient or visitor.

A hazard may also involve equipment or fabric of a building which has become unsafe.

BIBLIOGRAPHY

DOH 1994 Aids/HIV-infected Health Care Workers: Guidance on the Management of Infected Health Care Workers. COI/HSSH JO2-2302AR

BSI 1994 Medical gloves for single use Pt 2 Specification for physical properties. BS EN 455-2. London, BSI

Cocroft A 1995 Hepatitis B Virus and Employment in the NHS. British Journal of Hospital Medicine. 53 (10) 484-485

Control of Substances Hazardous to Health Regulations 1988

Dakin M J Yentis S M 1998 Latex Allergy : a strategy for management. Anaesthesia. 53. 774-781

Foley K 1993 Occupational exposure to trace anaesthetics. Quantifying the Risk. Journal of American Association of Nurse Anaesthetists. 61 (4)

Food Safety Act 1995

HSE 1997 A step by step guide to COSHH assessments. HSG(G) 97 ISBN 0-11-886379-7

HSE 1996 Electrical Safety and You. ISBN 0 7176 1207 4

Health and Safety at Work Act 1974

Health and Safety Commission Health Services Advisory Committee Guidance. Guidance on Manual Handling of Loads in the Health Services. ISBN 0-11-886354-1

HSE 1992 Manual Handling Operations Regulations. ISBN 0-717-60-411X

HSE 1994 New and Expectant Mothers at Work: a Guide for Employers, ref HS(G) 122, ISBN 0-7176-0826-3

HSE 1994 VDUs : An easy guide to the regulations. HS(G) 90 ISBN 0-7176-0735-6

HSE 1996 RIDDOR '96

HSE 1997 Infection risks to new and expectant mothers in the workplace: A guide for employers. ISBN 0-7176-1360-7

HSE Management of Health and Safety at Work. Approved Code of Practice: Management of Health and Safety at Work Regulations Ref L21 ISBN 0-7176-0412-8

MDA 1996 Latex sensitisation in the Health Care Setting. DB 9601

MDA 1997 Code of practice

NATN 1998 Safeguards for Invasive Procedures : the Management of Risks. Harrogate, NATN

NHS Executive 1996 Risk Management in the NHS. London, DOH

Recommendations for Inclusion in Local Policy

Good health and safety practice will encompass and provide protocols and procedures on the following:

1. Health and safety officer
2. Identification and documentation of incidents
3. Decontamination of equipment for repair
4. Preventative maintenance programmes
5. Medical gases and volatile agents in the perioperative setting
6. Noise
7. Stress
8. Manual handling operations
9. Control of Substances Hazardous to Health (COSHH)
10. Electrical equipment
11. Sharps
12. Care of pregnant staff
13. Floors, cleanliness, condition etc
14. Footwear
15. Clinical waste
16. Catering within the perioperative environment.

1. Health and safety officer

a. A health and safety officer must be appointed in every operating department. It is essential that this officer is trained for and understands his or her role and is allowed to fulfil the necessary duties.

b. All members of staff:

   i. Should know who their health and safety officer is.

   ii. Be aware of the role of the health and safety officer.

   iii. Receive training on the responsibilities of the employer and the employee in relation to health and safety.

   iv. Take an active part or be aware of the need and necessity for the updating of policies.

2. Identification and documentation of accidents and incidents of dangerous occurrences

a. All accidents to, or all incidents involving staff and/or equipment and buildings must be reported to the Head of Department and relevant paperwork completed in line with national guidelines (RIDDOR 1996).

b. The member of staff, if necessary, should seek medical assessment of any injury sustained. Local reporting protocols should be adhered to and all the documentation should go to an agreed central collecting point and a photocopy kept within the department.

c. A manager may initiate an internal enquiry into incidents where a problem has been identified. The use of incident reports is a valuable tool in development of protocols and procedures.

3. Decontamination of equipment for repair

Companies and medical equipment maintenance services require a certificate of decontamination of equipment sent for repair or returned from loan. The relevant paperwork should include:

a. Type, make and serial number of instrument or machine.

b. Name of department or hospital sending the equipment and a contact number.

c. The method of decontamination used e.g. steam sterilisation.

d. The name of the person responsible for sending the equipment for repair.

4. Preventative maintenance programmes

a. The employer has a responsibility for implementing a planned maintenance programme agreed between the Estates Service Department and the users/heads of department or the company from where the equipment was purchased or leased, (possibly with joint responsibility). The programme should cover all types of equipment.

b. Written documentation must be completed and signed by the senior member of staff which allows for maintenance to be carried out on areas of the perioperative environment and it's equipment, i.e. permit to work.

c. All items for repair must be separated from use, wherever possible being removed from the working environment and clearly labelled for repair.

5. Medical gases and volatile agents in the perioperative environment

It is essential that an employer has a policy outlining responsibilities and precautions necessary for the safe storage, handling and incidental exposure to medical gases and volatile agents.

a. The storage and use of cylinders.

b. The changing of cylinders.

c. Checking procedures after maintenance or work carried out on medical gas lines and equipment used in the delivery of medical gases and vapours.

d. Measures to reduce the occupational exposure to pollutants which should include scavenging systems designed to conduct expired gases and agents away from the occupational environment. Records should be kept of the monitoring levels in the perioperative environment.

e. There should be clear evidence of risk assessments, a spillage policy and training for staff dealing with volatile anaesthetic agents.

6. Noise

It is the employers responsibility to reduce so far as is reasonably practicable the employees exposure to noise. Refurbishment programmes, buildings works, extensions should be undertaken at such times when patient care is at a minimum.

7. Stress

Working in a perioperative environment can be extremely stressful. This is due to a number of factors including:

a. The constant updating and availability of technical equipment.

b. The pressure and type of work.

c. Unfavourable environmental conditions e.g. inappropriate temperature, humidity of the environment or a lack of natural light.

d. There is a potential risk that an employee who works excessively long hours, unsuitable shifts or on-calls, may encounter physical or mental ill health, or precipitate fatigue induced accidents or injury. There is therefore a need for adequate intervals for meals and rest as agreed within local policy. N.B. There are implications for this with the implementation of the European Working Time Directive.

8. Manual handling operations

a. A clear manual handling policy should exist within the organisation in accordance with the Manual Handling Operations Regulations (HSE) 1992.

b. Regular mandatory training in the correct methods of handling loads specific to the work area must be available to all staff:

i. During induction.

ii. And on a regular basis, at least annually in accordance with local policy.

iii. Clear attendance records must be maintained.

c. Trained risk assessors must be appointed identifying hazardous loads and identifying handling methods that eliminate or reduce risks to employees.

d. 'On the job' training may be demonstrated but formal instruction should be given by people who are themselves qualified to supply relevant information in these procedures. e.g. physiotherapists or ergonomic advisors.

e. The employer has a responsibility to supply sufficient manual handling aids that will reduce the risks to employees and patients.

f. The system should be in place to ensure that staff are adhering to the recommendations as laid down in local policy.

9. Control of Substances Hazardous to Health (COSHH)

The first duty of every employer is to prevent the exposure of the employee to substances hazardous to health.

a. The employer must ensure that adequate control has been secured in the first instance by:

i. Ensuring that all substances are COSHH assessed in line with local guidelines.

ii. Minimising the potential for exposure to hazardous substances by removal or using suitable alternatives.

iii. Measures other than personal protective equipment, e.g. the enclosure of the process

vi. The use of local exhaust ventilation, e.g. during the preparation of bone cement.

b. Subsequently the employer is charged with the provision of adequate supplies of suitable personal protective equipment, e.g. latex gloves, aprons, goggles.

The use of latex gloves has increased along with awareness of the need for the use of universal precautions. Guidelines for the use of latex gloves in terms of latex sensitisation must be adhered to.

c. It is the employers responsibility to ensure that staff have been informed of all hazardous substances within their working environment, with the identification of procedures to ensure control and prevention of injury from such substances. This should include methods of use and disposal.

d. Employers must ensure that there is a policy for the correct labelling and identification of containers used for hazardous substances.

e. All staff must be aware of procedures to be carried out in the event of injury related to such substances and the equipment for the same should be to hand at all times.

10. Electrical equipment

The provision and use of electrical equipment within the perioperative setting should comply within the recommendation of the Medical Devices Agency Code of Practice 1997 and therefore should:

a. Be checked by authorised designated personnel on delivery and before use.

b. Be used in accordance with the manufacturers recommendations.

c. Only be used by the employee who has been instructed in the use of setting up of that equipment, e.g. diathermy (monopolar, bi-polar, etc).

d. Have a planned preventative maintenance programme including a regular maintenance contract.

e. Ensure that all on loan or trial electrical equipment has a current certificate of indemnity and checks are carried out prior to its use.

11. Sharps

It is recommended that there must a strict policy for the disposal of sharps which includes the following statements:

a. Sharps containers should meet British Standard 7320.

b. Needles should not be re-sheathed.

c. Used needles and syringes should not be parted but placed as a whole in a yellow sharps bin or other recommended container in accordance with HSC specifications.

d. Special care should be taken when disposing of needles used to 'draw up' solutions for injections.

e. Sharps bins are to be sealed and sent for incineration when they are three quarters full.

f. Needles, blades and other sharps should be collected and contained safely during surgical procedures.

g. All staff should be made aware of the protocols to be followed in the event of a sharps injury.

h. The number, frequency and types of sharps injuries should be reviewed periodically.

12. Care of pregnant staff

a. If an employee suspects that she is pregnant, it is recommended that she reports this to her head of department and seeks confirmation from her GP.

b. If pregnant an employee should discuss occupational implications with the GP, occupational health advisor and/or head of department.

c. Certain activities may expose a developing foetus to risks. Therefore, consideration of pregnant staff is integral to risk assessments carried out on all activities and substances in the perioperative environment.

Risks that need consideration:

a) Ergonomic

i. The only restrictions likely during the first 20 weeks are to avoid excessive working hours.

ii. During pregnancy the woman's changing shape may affect aspects of her safety such as her ability to wear personal protective equipment, where the work involves sitting or standing for long periods or moving loads, re-allocation of duties may be required.

b) Infection

Provided that vaccinations are up to date, few additional precautions are necessary. Lengthy contact with patients being investigated or treated for known systemic infections should be avoided.

c) Radiation

Radiological and nuclear protection advisers must be consulted about particular areas where there are increased risks to a pregnant employee, re-allocation of duties may be required.

d) Chemical

Those substances which have maximum or occupational exposure limit should be assessed for use by and exposure to pregnant staff, extra precautions may be necessary.

e) Anaesthetics

All theatres should have local scavenging systems to recover anaesthetic gases\agents and ventilation systems should be in place to help prevent atmospheric pollution at all times. Recovery areas, anaesthetic rooms and minor theatres are usually smaller and therefore higher concentrations of waste gases\agents are found. It is recommended that exposure to waste anaesthetic gases be avoided, particularly during the first twelve weeks of pregnancy.

13. Floors, cleanliness, etc.

a. All floors must be kept clear of loose materials and prevented from becoming slippery. All reasonably practicable steps must be taken. Specific dangers are:

i. Spillage of water around scrub up area.

ii. Water spillage from autoclaves.

iii. Cables trailing on floors should be avoided, where this is unavoidable, these should be orange in colour and easily visible.

b. Approved notices should be in place which identify potential hazards, e.g. floor cleaning or spillages.

14. Footwear

This must be of correct fitting, conforming to non-slip requirement and be fully protective.

15. Clinical Waste

Clinical waste is considered to be:

a. Any waste which consists of wholly or partly of human or animal tissue, blood, body fluids, excretions, pharmaceutical products, swabs or dressings.

b. Any other waste arising from medical, nursing, pharmaceutical or similar practice which may cause infection to any person coming into contact with it.

Bags for the disposal\storage of clinical waste should be yellow and clearly marked 'clinical waste for incineration only'. These yellow bags should contain nothing but clinical waste. All staff who are required to handle bags of clinical waste should

i. Check that bags are effectively sealed.

ii. Handle bags by the neck only.

iii. Know the procedure in case of spillage.

iv. Ensure the origin of the waste is clearly marked.

v. Ensure that bags are closed when three quarters full only.

vi. Ensure the bags are intact prior to despatch.

vii. Ensure clinical waste is segregated from other types of waste.

16. Catering within the perioperative environment

If catering is available within the environment, it is essential that the requirements of the Food Safety Act 1995 are met.

Principles of Safe Practice in The Perioperative Environment

Management - *Section 5*

Reviewers

Jan Howells-Johnson RGN ONC ENB 998 925(1)
Education Committee NATN
Senior Sister Theatres
East Glamorgan Hospital

Kate Woodhead RGN DMS
National Vice Chairman NATN
Operating Theatre Manager
Leeds General Infirmary

Penny Gale RGN SCM IMSM Cert.
Operating Theatre Manager
Southampton General Hospital

Mike Fealey RGN
Theatre Manager
East Glamorgan Hospital

Kate Greaves RGN Cert Ed. DMS
Assistant Director Development and Training until March 98
Addenbrookes Hospital

Contributor

Sue Vincent RGN RM MA
National Chairman NATN
Senior Nurse Capital & Service Planning
West Suffolk Hospital

Principles of Safe Practice in
The Perioperative Environment

Management - *Section 5*

ETHICAL ISSUES

Introduction

The scope of ethical issues pertinent to perioperative care is vast. The main topics of concern are identified in this section and a bibliography is provided in order that the individual can become familiar with the wide range of moral and ethical dilemmas apparent in patient care, relationships with professional colleagues and research.

At its' most basic, the study of **ethics** is concerned with the meaning of such words as right, wrong, good, bad, ought and duty. It is concerned with the basis on which people, individually or collectively, decide that certain actions are right or wrong, and whether one ought to do something or has a right to do something (Rumbold 1993).

Advances in medical science create many ethical dilemmas for which there are no precedents. Perioperative practitioners are required to understand the moral responsibility that they have to their patients, their patients' families and to the nursing professional as a whole. The perioperative nurse must question his or her own moral and cultural beliefs, face their own fears and confront societal value systems. This can be emotionally demanding and often stresses ones' support systems but, with reflection and education, it can also be very rewarding.

All nurses are provided with a framework for moral and ethical decision making in the UKCC Code of Professional Conduct (1992), which sets out the essence of professional behaviour. Guidelines for Professional Practice (1996) expands on the sections of the Code of Conduct and offers a range of advice on interpretation of the Code with particular guidance on some of the many ethical and moral dilemmas faced by practising nurses.

Hospital trusts, private healthcare, and a variety of settings where perioperative care is delivered, have policy guidance which may have been developed nationally by professional organisations, local committees or be indicated by legislation. In addition, the Code of Professional Conduct makes all nurses responsible for understanding and applying to their practice all and any relevant guidance and to make judgements based on these. It is therefore essential for every nurse to use, reflect on and be conversant with the Code of Conduct and documents such as Guideline for Professional Practice. The Code of Conduct also indicates that every nurse should maintain and improve their professional knowledge and competence.

The Code of Conduct specifies that each registered nurse shall act, at all times in such a manner as to:

   i.   Safeguard and promote the interests of individual patients and clients.

   ii.   Serve the interests of society.

   iii.   Justify public trust and confidence.

   iv.   Uphold and enhance the good standing and reputation of the profession.

Clearly the Code identifies that within the value base of the profession decisions made by the individual nurse, should reflect, moral and ethical decision making within this framework. Perioperative nurses may experience ethical dilemmas in the course of their work particularly in areas such as those arising from the patient's rights of self determination; those arising in caring for patients and those resulting from the allocation of scarce resources. Practitioners and managers should ensure that opportunities for discussion, debate and reflection enable the development of analysis and critical thinking, in order to provide a comfortable working environment to promote ethical decision making.

When engaging in ethical decision making as an individual, as a team or an organisation it should also be recognised that some dilemmas have no "right" answers. No one solution will satisfy everyones' sense of right and wrong, so it is valuable to recognise that an approach which permits people to reach decisions that reflect compassion, respect, justice and recognise human fallibility is appropriate.

Conscientious Objection

Refusing to be involved in the care of patients because of their condition, sexual orientation, lifestyle or behaviour is unacceptable. The UKCC expects all registered practitioners to be non judgmental when providing care. Clause 7 of the Code of Conduct states that every nurse shall recognise and respect the uniqueness and dignity of each patient and respect their need for care, irrespective of the ethnic origin, religious beliefs, personal attributes and the nature of their health problems or any other factor.

There are circumstances in which practitioners, due to personal moral or religious beliefs, may not wish to be involved in certain types of treatments or care. The Code of Conduct states that individuals may "report to an appropriate person or authority, any conscientious objection which may be relevant to professional practice".

In law, nurses have the right to conscientiously object to take part in care in two specific areas. These are the Abortion Act 1967 (Scotland, England and Wales) which gives nurses the right to refuse to take part in an abortion, and the Human Fertilisation and Embryology Act 1990, which allows one the right to refuse to participate in technological procedures to achieve conception and pregnancy.

Research

Where the perioperative nurse is involved in research it is essential that the sponsor of the research and those participating have a clear understanding of their mutual obligations and responsibilities.

Any research carried out in the operating department must be necessary and contribute to further knowledge. All research proposals must be vetted and approved by an Ethics Committee and be in accordance with local policy.

Clinical Effectiveness

Increasing demands and advances in medical science are pressuring all healthcare professionals to examine current practice. Staff have a professional duty to keep up with innovations and maintain the balance of increasing workloads. There is an emerging focus on clinical effectiveness and evidence based care which indicates that there are many challenges to providing effective and cost efficient services to patients within a structured and accountable framework.

Education in nursing and nursing professionalism are developing an increased recognition that nurses need evidence that their care procedures are based on fact and not tradition, and can be shown to be cost effective. Castledine (1997) says evidence based nursing must always maintain a balance between research on a clinical subject and information gained from the patient.

The shift in practice from one that is based on tradition to one that is based on evidence is bound to be a difficult one for nursing (Hicks 1997, Simpson 1996). Cullum (1996) identifies that this is because nurses working in clinical practice are constrained by the reality of action taking precedence over reflection.

Perioperative nurses need to develop individual strategies to overcome these challenges and use research findings to advance the art and science of perioperative nursing practice.

Techniques already widely in use by perioperative nurses may encourage those wishing to enhance and develop their evidence based care by using:

i. Reflective practice.

ii. Audit, nursing and collaborative feedback.

iii. Individual performance review.

iv. Quality circles.

v. Team briefings.

The environment and culture of the department should support individual practitioners to implement evidence based care.

Clinical Supervision

The implementation of clinical supervision is now seen as a critical element in the provision of safe and accountable practice (Faugier 1995).

Clinical supervision is a formal arrangement that enabled nurses to discuss their work regularly with another experienced professional (Kohner 1994).

The professional fulfilling the supervisory role is most likely to be a nurse. The relevance of his or her supervisory skills and the relevance of his or her experience and expertise to the needs of the person receiving supervision is more important than their seniority or professional group.

Clinical supervision involves reflecting on practice in order to learn from experience and improve competence. It is the development of insight into ones' own practice.

The UKCC states that clinical supervision is not a "managerial control system" although some nurses may believe that the use of the word supervision indicates some hierarchical function. Clinical supervision is therefore a professional relationship between a supervisor and surpervisee that is grounded in the idea of joint responsibility and ownership, each partner giving equally in terms of commitment and open, honest discussion (Farrington 1995).

Risk Management

Risk management is the methodology used to identify, assess and take action to reduce risks.

Healthcare organisations have a corporate responsibility to provide risk management strategies to protect the public and employees from harm.

Operating departments are recognised as areas having high risk potential and it is the responsibility of staff to be vigilant in identifying and reporting issues of concern. The process of risk identification and management of those risks is the responsibility of every practitioner. The environment and culture of the department should encourage individual practitioners to challenge poor practice and take action accordingly.

Individual practitioners must be committed to management of potential risks to patients, visitors and colleagues. Department guidelines should enable practitioners to clearly identify and report sources of potential risk. Regular monitoring and audit of practice must be undertaken and the outcomes reviewed within the multi-disciplinary team.

Education and training issues for staff resulting from risk management audit and documentation must be undertaken regularly.

Integrated Care Pathways

Integrated Care pathways may also be known as Critical Care pathways and Clinical Care Pathways.

Care pathways are identified as an approach which specifies key activities by different professionals on a continuum to produce the best achievable outcomes for an episode of care.

The care pathway is ideally an outcome of the collaboration at specified stages of care, between members of the multidisciplinary team, to assess, plan, implement and evaluate individual care.

It is recommended that there is access to a database or information source which allows staff immediate, updated and relevant information in support of evidence based practice. For this reason, to be fully effective it needs to be sited within the operating department.

BIBLIOGRAPHY

Abortion Act 1967 (Scotland, England and Wales)

Dimond B 1990 Legal Aspects of Nursing. London, Prentice Hall

Hind M 1997 Clarifying accountability in operating theatre practice. Nursing Standard. 12 (3) 44-45

Human Fertilisation and Embryology Act 1990

NATN 1997 Developing New Roles for Non-Medical Staff within Perioperative Care. Harrogate, NATN

Tingle J 1997 Expanded role of the Nurse: accountability confusion. British Journal of Nursing. 6 (17) 1011-1013

UKCC 1992 Code of Professional Conduct. (3rd edition) London, UKCC

UKCC 1992 The Scope of Professional Practice. London, UKCC

UKCC 1996 Guidelines for Professional Practice. London, UKCC

Ethics

Rumbold G 1993 Ethics in Nursing Practice. (2nd Edition) London, Bailliere Tindall

UKCC 1992 Code of Professional Conduct. (3rd edition) London, UKCC

UKCC 1996 Guidelines for Professional Practice. London, UKCC

Clinical Effectiveness

Castledine G 1997 Evidence based nursing, where is the evidence? British Journal of Nursing. 6 (5) 290

Hicks C 1997 The Dilemma of incorporating research into Clinical Practice. British Journal of Nursing. 6 (9) 511-515

Simpson B 1996 Evidence based nursing practice; The State of the Art. Canadian Nurse. 92 (10) 22-25

Cullum N Sheldon T 1996 Clinically challenged (evidence based healthcare and research and availability to nurses). Nursing Management. 3 (4) 14-16

Faugier J Butterworth T 1995 Clinical Supervision, a position paper. School of Nursing Studies, University of Manchester

Clinical Supervision

Farrington A 1995 Defining and setting the parameters of clinical supervision. British Journal of Nursing. 4 (15) 874-875

Kohner N 1994 Clinical Supervision in Practice. London, King's Fund Centre

UKCC 1996 Position statement on clinical supervision for nursing and health visiting. London, UKCC

Integrated Care Pathways

Johnson S 1995 Pathway to the heart of care quality. Nursing Management. 1 (8) 26-27

Wigfield A Boon E 1996 Critical care pathways development: the way forward. British Journal of Nursing. 5 (12) 723-725

Further Reading

The NHS Confederation 1997 Acting on the Evidence progress in the NHS Health Services Management Centre, Birmingham

Welsh Office   1995 Towards Evidence Based Practice
               1995 Improving Access to Evidence and Information
               1996 Helping Practitioners Use the Evidence
               1996 Developing the Working Environment

NHS Executive 1996 Promoting Clinical Effectiveness
               1996 Clinical Guidelines
               1996 Clinical Audit in the NHS
               1998 Clinical Effectiveness: A resource pack

Allitt Enquiry 1994 Clinical Supervision for Nursing and Health Visiting Professions. London, DOH

Benjamin M and Curtis J 1992 Ethics in Nursing. (3rd Edition) Oxford, Oxford University Press.

Dimond B 1995 Legal Aspects of Nursing Practice. (2nd Edition) London, Hall

Dixon E 1984 The Theatre Nurse and the Law. London, Croom Helm

Mardell A 1996 Advocacy : Exploring the concept. British Journal of Theatre Nursing. 6 (7) 34-36.1

NATN 1995 Risk Assessment Guidelines (RAG). Harrogate, NATN

Pyne R 1992 Professional Discipline in Nursing, Midwifery and Health Visiting. Oxford, Blackwell Scientific

Tingle J, Cribb A 1995 Nursing Law and Ethics. Oxford, Blackwell Scientific

Tschudin V 1994 Ethics and Nursing. The Caring Relationship. (2nd Edition) Oxford, Butterworth Heinemann

Spinks M 1996 Risk Assessments : is there a risk? British Journal of Theatre Nursing. 6 (7) 32-33

Accountability

The United Kingdom Central Council for Nurses, Midwives and Health Visiting have developed a number of publications which give registered nurse practitioners guidance in their practice in order to protect the public.

NATN recommends that every nurse becomes familiar with the documents and uses them to guide accountability and decision making in their practice. Operating department focus groups may wish to include professional issues in their regular discussions.

Issues which regularly concern perioperative nurses, and which are raised for professional guidance are:

    i.   The role of the RGN in the multidisciplinary team.

    ii. Accepting delegated responsibilities.

    iii. Delegating responsibilities.

    iv. Developing personal practice.

    v. Challenging poor practice.

Accountability is an integral part of professional practice, as in the course of practice the nurse has to make judgements in a wide variety of circumstances. Accountability is fundamentally concerned with weighing up the interests of patients in complex situations, using professional knowledge, judgement and skills to make a decision for which the practitioner can account. As a concept, accountability may be relatively easy to define, but in practice it can often be difficult for practitioners to understand fully

how, why and when they may be called to account for their actions or omissions (Hind 1997).

Every registered practitioner holds a position of responsibility on whom other people may reply. The practitioner is professionally accountable to the UKCC, as well as having a contractual accountability to their employer and accountability to the law for action.

Accountability to self:

Dimond (1990) states that self accountability is the moral dimension which cannot be legally enforced, although it is argued that it is at the heart of best professional competence and skill.

Legal Accountability:

This mode of accountability involves being accountable to the public through criminal law and the criminal courts and fortunately in healthcare is relatively uncommon, but litigation for negligence through civil action in the courts is increasing alarmingly.

Contractual Accountability:

This involves the relationship between the registered nurse and the employer, and is based on the individuals' contract of employment and the job description.

Professional Accountability:

The principles of professional accountability are set out in the Code of Professional Conduct published by the statutory body The United Kingdom Central Council (UKCC) which regulates in law the actions of nurses, midwives and health visitors in order to protect the interest of patients and public.

The Code of Conduct sets out the context of that accountability. It begins with the statement that:

"Each registered nurse, midwife and health visitor shall act, at all times, in such a manner as to: safeguard and promote the interests of individual patients and clients; serve the interests of society; justify public trust and confidence and uphold and enhance the good standing of the professions".

Each clause of the code begins with the statement that:

"As a registered nurse, midwife or health visitor, you are personally responsible for your practice and, in the exercise of your professional accountability, must...."

To assist individual registered practitioners working in perioperative practice with the way in which the Code of Conduct can guide them through some of their dilemmas, the previous examples of commonly expressed problems have been referenced to specific clauses of the Code.

Role of the RGN in the multidisciplinary team

The Code refers the practitioner to Clause 6 which states that as a registered nurse... you must.."work in a collaborative and co-operative manner with health care professionals and others involved in providing care, and recognise and respect their particular contributions within the care team"; and Clause 14, "assist professional colleagues, in the context of your own knowledge, experience and sphere of responsibility, to develop their professional competence and assist others in the care team including informal carers, to contribute safely and to a degree appropriate to their roles".

Delegation

The practitioner is referred to Clause 2 of the Code of Conduct which states that you must..."ensure that no act or omission on your part, or within your sphere of responsibility, is detrimental to the interest, condition or safety of patients and clients"

and

if work is delegated to someone who is not registered with UKCC, the nurses' accountability is to ensure that the person who does the work is able to do it and that appropriate levels of supervision or support are in place.

The Scope of Professional Practice (UKCC 1992) section 22 and 23 specify that "registered nurses... must remain accountable for ... standards of care and determining the activity of their support staff", and that "health care assistants must not be allowed to work beyond their level of competence.

Developing Personal Practice

Clause 3 and 4 of the Code of Conduct state that you must..."maintain and improve your professional knowledge and competence" and "acknowledge any limitations in your knowledge and competence and decline any duties or responsibilities unless able to perform them in a safe and skilled manner".

The practitioner should also be familiar with the Scope of Professional Practice (UKCC 1992).

Accepting Delegation

The practitioner is referred to Clause 4 which states that you must "acknowledge any limitations in your knowledge and competence and decline any duties and responsibilities unless able to perform them in a safe and skilled manner".

Challenging Poor Practice

Clause 11 states that the practitioner must..."report to an appropriate person or authority, having regard to physical, psychological and social effect on patients and clients, and circumstances in the environment of care which could jeopardise standards of practice" and in addition, Clause 12 states that the practitioner must..."report to an appropriate person or authority any circumstances in which safe and appropriate care for patients and clients cannot be provided".

Confidentiality

Clause 10 clearly states that the practitioner must... "protect all confidential information concerning patients and clients obtained in the course of professional practice and make disclosures only with consent, where required by the order of a Court or where you can justify disclosure in the wider public interest".

Scope of Professional Practice

The practice of nursing, midwifery and health visiting requires the application of knowledge and the simultaneous exercise of judgement and skill. Practice takes place in a context of continuing change and development. Such change and development may result from advances in research leading to improvements in treatment and care, from alterations to the provision of health and social services care or as a result of new approaches to professional practice. Practice must, therefore, be sensitive to the needs of individual patients and clients and have the capacity to adjust, where and when appropriate, to changing circumstances.

The scope of professional practice refers to the range of responsibilities which fall to individual nurses, midwives and health visitors related to their personal experience, education and skill.

The education which every nurse receives prior to initial registration cannot effectively meet the changing and complex demands of the range of modern healthcare. So it can be seen that just as practice must remain dynamic, sensitive, relevant and responsive to the changing needs of patients, so too must education for practice. Post registration equips practitioners with additional and more specialist skills necessary to meet the special needs of patients.

Within the Code of Professional Conduct, the relevant clauses of the code which relate to the scope of professional practice are:

"As a registered nurse, midwife or health visitor you are personally accountable for your practice and, in the exercise of your professional accountability, must:

i. Act always in such a manner as to promote and safeguard the interests and well being of patients and clients.

ii. Ensure that no act or omission on your part, or within your sphere of responsibility, is detrimental to the interests, condition or safety of patients and clients.

iii. Maintain and improve your professional knowledge and competence.

iv. Acknowledge any limitations in your knowledge and competence and decline any duties or responsibilities unless able to perform them in a safe and skilled manner.

It is recommended that copies of the Scope of Professional Practice and The Code of Conduct are available as a resource in the Operating Department. Copies are available from UKCC.

Developing Roles

New roles are developing in perioperative care which has led to some confusion surrounding the lines of accountability, particularly where nurses are carrying out care which would have previously been undertaken by medical personnel. There is considerable professional freedom for development of roles which cross traditional lines of demarcation between the professions, provided that the three areas of obligation, to regulatory bodies, to civil law and to employment law are observed. Appropriate educational and managerial safeguards should be in place and role development proceed by negotiation and agreement amongst the professions concerned.

However, these changes raise important legal issues particularly with regard to apparently conflicting guidance on delegation of medical procedures performed by non medically qualified health professionals and ambiguities remain unresolved. Practitioners are referred to "Developing New Roles for Non-Medical Staff Within Perioperative Care" (NATN 1997).

For post holders of newly developing roles in the operating department, whether registered nurses or members of other disciplines such as ODPs' obligation to civil employment law will be similar. But there will be differences in respect of obligation to professional regulatory bodies.

Operating Department Practitioners

Operating department assistants/practitioners work closely within perioperative care settings with nurses. It is often incorrectly stated that ODA/Ps are not accountable for their actions because they do not currently have professional regulation in the way nurses do. The professional association for ODPs, the Association for Operating Department Practitioners, (formerly British Association for Operating Department Assistants) currently operates a voluntary register, and despite a protracted campaign for professional regulation, it is not yet formally established (Hind 1997).

Principles of Safe Practice in The Perioperative Environment

Management - *Section 5*

DEPARTMENTAL ORGANISATION

Introduction

Effective organisation is essential to the efficient running of an operating department.

Operating departments may be comprised of single, twin or multi-theatre, with or without support services. Methods of organisation will vary according to the design and management structure of each department.

Since the early 1990s, a number of government initiatives have affected departmental organisation to ensure that resources are managed effectively and information is gathered against the Patient's Charter criteria; in addition, the contracting system has asked difficult, but important, questions of health care providers. These initiatives have challenged the traditional role of operating department management and have demanded a change to an internal responsive service thus ensuring effective capacity planning and scheduling linked to the supply of staff and equipment. These requirements of efficiency and effectiveness apply to all operating departments whether these are in the public or independent sectors.

Operating department managers need to be involved therefore, with all stages of the planning process as it affects the individual and collective surgical patient and ensure that they receive the necessary timely information about workload. The principles of process management far from depersonalising the care of patients can ensure that each patient is treated as an individual and that they receive their anaesthetic and/or surgical intervention at the most appropriate time for the best result.

Operating department managers have a responsibility to identify how their department supports the strategic direction of the main organisation, developing a departmental strategy statement and annual objectives which are understood and their achievement supported by all operating department staff.

In addition, operating department managers now function within general management or directorate structures requiring close co-operation between, and communications with, business managers and clinical directors.

BIBLIOGRAPHY

Johnson M 1994 Planning Operating Departments an Evolution. British Journal of Theatre Nursing. 4 (7) 14-15

Lewis M 1994 Communication in theatres. Surgical Nurse. 7 (1) 27-29

NATN 1994 Quality Assessment Document. (QUAD) Harrogate, NATN

NATN 1995 Risk Assessment Guide. (RAG) Harrogate, NATN

NATN 1998 Good Employment Practice. Principles of Safe Practice in the Perioperative Environment. Harrogate, NATN

NHS Estates 1991 Health Building Note 26 Operating Departments. London, HMSO

NHS Estates 1991 Health Building Note 27 Intensive Therapy Unit. London, HMSO

NHS Estates 1993 Health Building Note 2 The Whole Hospital Briefing and Operational Policies. London, HMSO

NHS Estate 1993 Health Building Note 13 Sterile Services Department. London, HMSO

NHS Estates 1993 Health Building Note 52: Vol 1
Accommodation for Day Care : Day Surgery Unit.
London, HMSO

NHS Estates 1994 Health Building Note 52: Vol 2
Accommodation for Day Care: Endoscopy Unit.
London, HMSO

NHS Estates 1995 Health Building Note 52: Vol 3
Accommodation for Day Care : Medical Investigation
and Treatment Unit. London, HMSO

NHS Estates 1997 Health Building Note 52: Sup 1 Day
Surgery : Review of Schedules of Accommodation.
London, HMSO

Recommendations for Inclusion in Local Policy

Areas for consideration will include design, communications and management control.

1. **Planning and Design of Facilities for Surgical Intervention.**

   a. Advances in surgery, anaesthetics and practice as a regular occurrence have made it necessary to review the facilities for operative procedures as part of the overall business planning process. However, whatever the developments, the main principles of design for operating departments are still applicable wherever surgical intervention takes place:

      i. The siting of the operating department will ensure optimum infection control and maximum efficiency.

      ii. The zoning of particular areas from outer (changing room) to inner cleaner areas (operating suite) is necessary.

      iii. It is recommended that patient flow should move from preoperative, to theatre, to postoperative area.

      iv. The delivery of supplies must be kept separate from patient areas.

      v. It is essential that there are safe and effective methods of disposal and collection of waste from clean and dirty areas of the department.

   b. Principles of the planning process are the same for any health care facility and should be applied to upgrades and refurbishments as well as new buildings. Key representatives of those involved with the day to day running of the facility must be part of the planning team, as well as a surgeon and anaesthetist, and must work closely with the design team to ensure that the department will be functional and can be utilised efficiently in line with local policy. Before the design team can begin their work the departmental operational policy must be reviewed and updated and the overall policy for the whole hospital taken into account, so that a brief can be prepared. This must identify the following:

      i. Space available and relationships to other areas and departments within the hospital.

      ii. Whole hospital policies that affect the management of the department.

      iii. Types of surgery to be undertaken and special technology required.

      iv. Policies and procedures for administration of anaesthesia.

      v. Post anaesthetic recovery policies and availability of high dependency and ICU beds.

      vi. General equipment requirements for each room or area.

      vii. Information technology systems to be used.

      viii. Average maximum number of patients

to be treated and the number of operating rooms required.

ix. Work flow.

x. Number of staff and the maximum number likely to be working in each of the areas at any one time; normal working hours; maximum number of theatres expected to be working at any one time within and out of normal working hours.

xi. Support services available within and outside the department.

c. The actual space required for each area is determined by the activity, equipment and number of staff required. Design guidance makes recommendations in relation to this; the minimum space recommended for an operating theatre today is 40 square meters, with a ceiling height of 3 metres to facilitate a main operating light and satellite. The factors that have the most significant impact on operating theatre design include:

i. The operating table, lights and lighting.

ii. Imaging and monitoring equipment.

iii. Anaesthetic techniques and associated technologies.

iv. Robotics.

v. Telemonitoring and education.

vi. Supply and disposal.

vii. Surgical instrumentation.

viii. Support services already available or required; surrounding areas, environment, logistics and management.

d. Zoning of different functions is still recommended, although with the development of more sophisticated ventilation systems such as the Ultra Clean,

which provides a zone virtually free from contamination with a minimum of 10 air changes per hour, it is probably only necessary for infection control purposes to restrict access to the actual theatre and sterile supply areas. With conventional ventilation systems, four access zones are identified:

i. A general or outer zone, including the reception and transfer, staff change and other areas that require access by hospital staff.

ii. A limited or clean zone for access by staff once they have changed into theatre clothing.

iii. A restricted zone for sterile supply, preparation areas, induction of anaesthetic and scrub up.

iv. An operative field for the surgical team only.

e. To facilitate all the functions necessary to enable surgical intervention to take place safely and efficiently, space is required for:

i. A staff room and changing area.

ii. Offices and a control base, reception and transfer incorporating porters base.

iii. A central store incorporating a sterile supply area.

iv. The operating suite, incorporating scrub up and preparation areas and utility room.

v. Administration of anaesthetic/preparation, post anaesthetic recovery.

vi. Disposal hold and collection base.

f. As well as the main principles outlined it is important that the facility is both functional and meets local needs related to policies and procedures. For facilities in the United Kingdom the design should be based on the principles outlined in the guidelines of the relevant Health Building Note published by NHS Estates in conjunction with the appropriate Health Technical Memoranda. These can be obtained from the Stationery Office Publications Centre, P.O. Box 276, London SW8 5DT, tel: 0171 873 9090, fax 0171 873 8200.

2. General Considerations

a. Design.

    i. The siting of the operating department will ensure optimum infection control and maximum efficiency and where possible, they should be sited near services, wards and intensive care units.

    ii. The zoning of particular areas from outer (changing rooms) to inner cleaner areas (theatre suite) is no longer considered microbiology essential, but it is recommended to support security and discipline.

    iii. It is recommended that patient flow should move from preoperative, to theatre, to postoperative.

    iv. The delivery of supplies must be kept separate from the patient entrance and exit areas.

    v. It is essential that there are safe and effective methods of disposal and collection of waste.

b. Communication

Effective internal and external communication across all members of the multi-disciplinary team plays a vital role in the smooth running of the operative department and supports the morale of staff. Consideration should be given therefore to:

    i. Methods of staff briefing and reporting, both written and verbal, through all grades, which should take place at regular intervals.

    ii. Liaison with medical staff to ensure that timely information about proposed workload, elective or emergency, is available to allow effective resource allocation.

    iii. Active communication with wards, which will include the development of the effective documentation related to patient care and quality issues.

    iv. Active communication with support services.

    v. The use of adequate telephone, intercom, bleep and call system in larger departments.

    vi. The skills and techniques of communication with patients during their stay in the operating department.

3. Management Considerations

There are three major aspects of organisational management which need to be applied across all areas of the operating department; these are strategic, tactical and operational.

a. Strategic

    i. Effective organisations develop a 3-5 year strategic plan which gives direction to the core and secondary roles of the organisation and which clarifies ongoing and new business developments.

    ii. Operating departments should reflect the overall strategy and identify specific developments by producing their own strategic direction statement and ensuring that this is published widely to all staff. When constructing a strategic planning document, the following areas require attention:

a) Philosophy statement which identifies the key role of the department and establishes the quality of care which can be expected for all patients and describes the working environment for staff.

b) Key objectives - such as:

Financial
Improvements against Major
Performance Indicators
Developments in Clinical Practice
Team Management
Education and Training
Research

All objectives must be written so that the outcomes are clearly defined and measurable and have dates for achievement.

b. Tactical

i. This involves the setting and agreeing of standards for the department as a whole and should be linked to the departmental strategic direction statement. These standards will relate to the quality of:

Care delivery
Information in order to assist the decision making
process (including that about patients, staff,
equipment theatre users)
Education and training

ii. Use of existing facilities (capacity planning), budgetary control and overall organisation of elective and emergency workload (demand scheduling) are all aspects which fall under the remit of tactical management.

iii. All objectives must be written so that the outcomes are clearly defined and measurable and have dates for achievement. Formal systems are essential for monitoring, evaluating and reviewing these standards.

c. Operational

Each operating department should have an up-to-date operational policy. This involves the setting and agreeing of standards which relate to the day to day function of the operating department in order to ensure a high quality service and safe practices. These standards should reflect the tactical outcomes and be written so that the outcomes are clearly defined and measurable with dates for achievement. They will relate to:

The cost of effective service delivery

Resource scheduling and allocation level of cancelled procedures (1%)

Demand scheduling and throughput use of emergency theatre during normal working hours maintaining agreed standards of theatre use.

Procedures and policies the collection of information the development of individuals and teams

4. **Topics for Development**

a. Patient Care

A quality assurance system to be operational includes the effect departmental procedures have on the overall surgical patient process, the Patients' Charter standards, standards for ensuring a safe environment and the maintenance of records and documentation.

b. Staff:

The operating department is a stressful and complex environment and the continuous recruitment and development of new staff is very costly. Therefore it is incumbent upon the operating department manager to ensure that effective support systems are in place in order to encourage the retention of staff. It will be necessary to include:

i. The observance of local policies, employment legislation and/or Whitley Council conditions of service.

ii. Job descriptions and person specifications for each grade of staff.

iii. Systems for monitoring, reviewing and evaluating workforce and utilisation.

iv. Personnel and occupational health procedures to ensure good employment practice.

v. An education and training programme which can be applied with equity for all staff.

vi. A system of individual performance review with associated individual development planning.

c. Activity:

It will be necessary to include:

i. Provision of suitable operating facilities for patients who are undergoing anaesthetic and/or surgery as in- or out-patients.

ii. Information describing the length of elective and emergency procedures which allows operating sessions to be planned and negotiated effectively.

iii. Communication pathways to ensure that prepared patients receive the expected procedure and arrive in the operating department in an optimum condition.

iv. Defined procedures for booking cases into scheduled and emergency systems with clear direction about the staff who must be involved.

v. Support for the decision making process, by clarifying the type of information required about operating department activity; for example:

  Patients cancellations
  Over-runs
  Under-runs
  Staff sickness levels
  High cost procedures

vi. Patient information systems can support the collection of data in the operating department and ensure the continuity of care and information for patients.

vii. A major incident plan.

d. Maintenance

Health care organisations have agreed programmes for maintaining the building and mechanical standards of the building with programmes for planned major plant repair and replacement. There must be systems to ensure that the fabric of the building and mechanical and electrical plant are maintained in good order and policies to ensure safe functioning of the mechanical and electrical installations in the operating department.

e. Equipment

Systems should be in place for the planned replacement of expensive items, for monitoring the purchase and maintenance of all equipment and for reporting ineffective or broken equipment. Standards must be set at an operational level for safe usage of equipment which must relate to the manufacturer's guidelines.

f. Consumables

Systems should be in place for enabling the purchase of an adequate and effective supply of consumables, for monitoring, evaluating and reviewing consumable supplies to ensure the maintenance of adequate and relevant stock levels and for ordering, receiving and storing supplies to maintain agreed stock levels.

g. Health and Safety

Health and Safety issues relating to the environment, staff and patients must be considered at all times. For further information refer to Good Employment Practice, Principles Of Safe Practice In The Perioperative Environment.

INDEX

T

U

V

W

NOTES